Dame Kelly Holmes

RUNNING

life

Mindset, fitness & nutrition for positive wellbeing

PHOTOGRAPHY BY PETER CASSIDY

KYLE BOOKS

An Hachette UK Company
www.hachette.co.uk

First published in Great Britain in 2018 by
Kyle Books, an imprint of Kyle Cathie Ltd
Carmelite House
50 Victoria Embankment
London EC4Y 0DZ
www.kylebooks.co.uk

ISBN: 978 0 85783 535 2

Mindset contributor: Tanya Wright and Fitness contributor: Alison Rose MCSP HCPC
Editor: Vicky Orchard
Design: Studio nic&lou
Photography: Peter Cassidy
Food styling and recipe development: Lizzie Harris
Props styling: Cynthia Blackett
Make-up: Emilie Walkden MUA
Production: Lisa Pinnell and Caroline Alberti

A Cataloguing in Publication record for this title is available from the British Library

Printed and bound in Italy

10 9 8 7 6 5 4 3 2 1

Contents

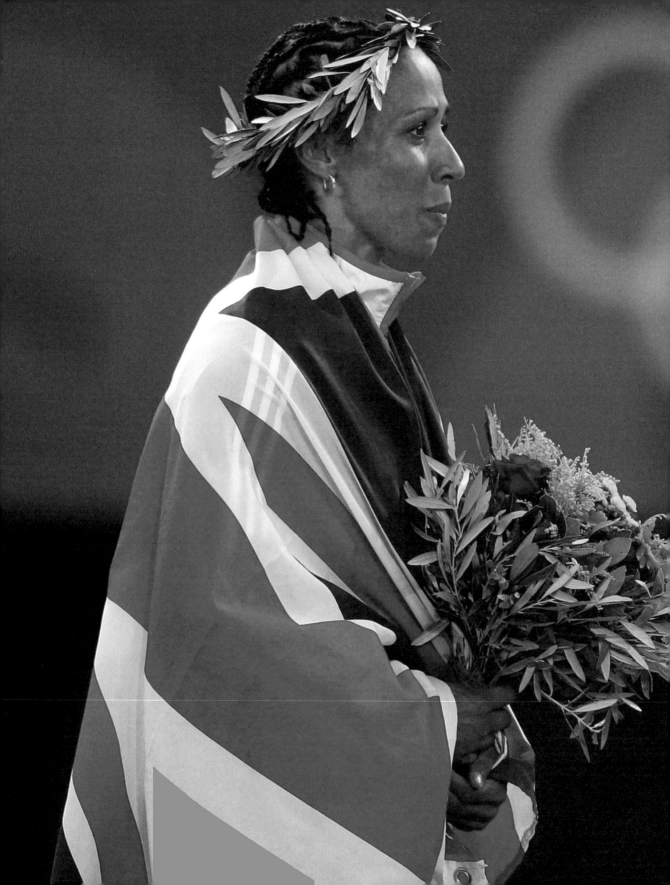

CHALLENGE
THE IMPOSSIBLE

I believe that things in life
are possible to achieve if,
firstly, you believe they are;

Secondly, you have a reason to
know it could be possible.

It's human nature that we only ever believe
we can achieve something if we have
been a whisper away from the outcome
in the past. However, through adventure,
inquisitive behaviour, determination,
focus and opportunity we can push
ourselves to be better than we
thought we could ever be.

introduction

WHAT IS MOTIVATED LIVING AND WHAT WILL THIS BOOK DO FOR YOU?

To me, motivated living means a determination to reach your full potential and be the best version of yourself in whatever you do. Being proud, positive and fulfilling your talent. It's about being motivated to learn, which comes from being driven, ambitious, inspired and determined. It's about feeling free to dream and to act on those dreams. We all need goals and hopes – my aim is that this book helps you to realise all of yours.

Every fitness or health professional has their own approach, different methods and their own version of what works for them. Buying my book is the first step to a healthier lifestyle that will help you feel physically and mentally at your peak. Whether you are taking the first tentative steps on your fitness journey, or looking for help to stay focused and maintain your mental and physical wellbeing, being the best version of yourself can be daunting and feel impossible at times. I want this book to show you that the magic triangle of nutrition, fitness and positive thinking is the key to a happier and healthier life. Life is not a rehearsal, it's real, it's a journey and it's yours, so the one thing you can achieve through reading this book is trying to be the best version of yourself.

My approach is not extreme and impossible, but making changes will need focus and commitment. Sometimes the biggest thing in your way is you and that is the first thing we will tackle. Since I was a young girl I always believed that no matter what barriers are put in your way, it is essential to find a path to overcoming them, however big or small. I can't really remember when I first started thinking: *'What's next? What am I here to do or to achieve?'* But it is how I try to think every day.

I set my goals pretty early in life and I had two main ones: from the age of 14 I wanted to be Olympic 1500m champion and in the British Army as a

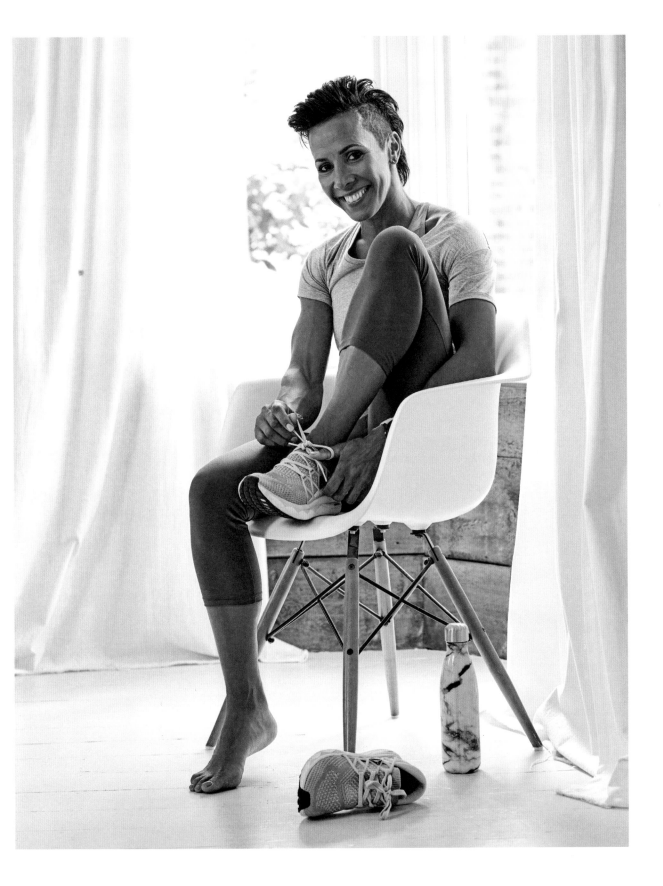

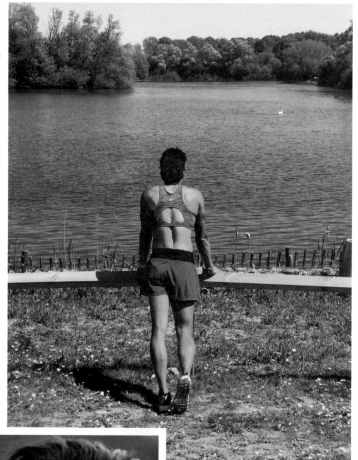

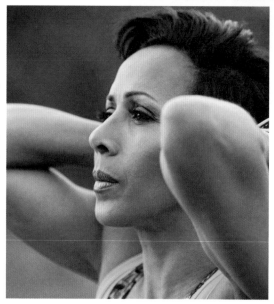

Be Strong. Be Positive.

I think I have a trait that is all about pushing to the next level and not taking no for an answer, but it isn't always easy.

Physical Training Instructor. I am proud to say I achieved both. The British Army brought out in me the same characteristics as sport. I think I have a trait that is all about pushing to the next level and not taking no for an answer, but it isn't always easy.

Over the years I have aspired to live in a motivated way, but life is complex and things are rarely as they seem on the outside. When I look back at my own achievements I can see that, to some people, I must have had it all. But I spent my early years torn between being driven and struggling to find my identity. The turning point came when a PE teacher spotted my talent for running and helped me believe that it was possible to be good at something. I started competing when I was 12 years old, so from an early age I had a determination to be the best. I hated losing but I learnt from my mistakes. I continued my junior international career until I was seventeen.

I then went on to join the British Army. I gave up my athletics to concentrate on my military career, in which I served for nine and half years as a sergeant. Leaving the army at the end of 1997, I then devoted myself full-time to athletics and to pursuing my dream of becoming an Olympic champion, which turned into a double gold medal-winning performance at the 2004 Athens Olympics. I achieved my dreams and worked hard at all that I did. Looking back I had an amazing career, unbeaten as a British athlete for 12 years and winning 12 major world-class medals. However, the demands on my mental health were huge and things weren't as perfect as they may have seemed.

I was winning medals around the world and, on the outside, that's an amazing feat, but on the inside, I didn't want to be here. Lots of sports people have ups and downs: you are terrified you will never achieve your dream, but it is having the dream that keeps you going and pushing for success. I adored everything about my sporting career but it is a complicated relationship and sometimes sport can be the loneliest place in the world: you can be surrounded by a team and still feel utterly alone. I felt like this for a long time but the wake-up call came when I couldn't see the end of the road or any light at all because of all the injuries I had. You can't explain or understand it unless you've dealt with it but depression is a dark place to be.

I think there are a lot of people who really don't know how best to tap into their inner confidence, but believing in yourself is vital if you want to achieve the very best out of life.

Our bodies are pretty amazing and our brain, in particular, is a magical, wonderful tool. But if something goes wrong you can be seriously derailed and it can be hard to recalibrate. When someone has a form of depression – in whatever form that takes (eating disorders, self-harming etc) – it is all about hurting. It's about having an issue to deal with and that issue is never the same for everyone.

I truly believe that the key to long-term mental and physical health is intervention – not with medication unless medical intervention is a last resort, but moving and fuelling your mind and body properly so that you don't have to try to avoid that dark place to begin with. We shouldn't wait until something terrible happens and then try to cure it, we should have the tools to nurture and take care of ourselves rather than relying on pills. Our bodies and minds are finely tuned machines and need careful feeding and maintaining. It isn't just about eating good food and getting fit, it is also about how you use fitness and nutrition as a way of feeling good and being better than you think you can be.

I think there are a lot of people who really don't know how best to tap into their inner confidence, but believing in yourself is vital if you want to achieve the very best out of life. It is about setting your sights high and realising there are three strands to excellence. What you feed your body feeds your mind and how you move your body enables both. I want this book to be about lifelong health and wellbeing, not a short-term transformation fuelled by panic as you look at the scales.

With that in mind, this book will be spilt into three sections: Mindset, Fitness and Nutrition. I talk openly about my own mental health struggles as well as giving you tips, fitness plans and delicious recipes. This is a way of life for me. Nothing is perfect and my struggles have changed me – but they have also given me focus and helped me to realise who I am. Essentially, I was a runner who learned to perform at the very highest level and that set me on my path. That path won't be the same for everyone – but I want you to know that, whatever your highest level is, this book can help you reach it.

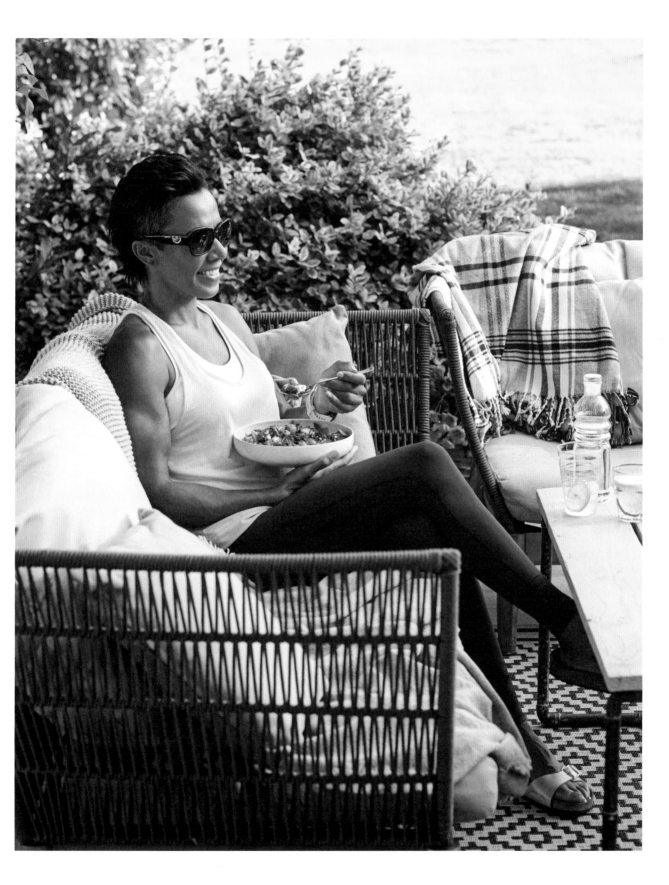

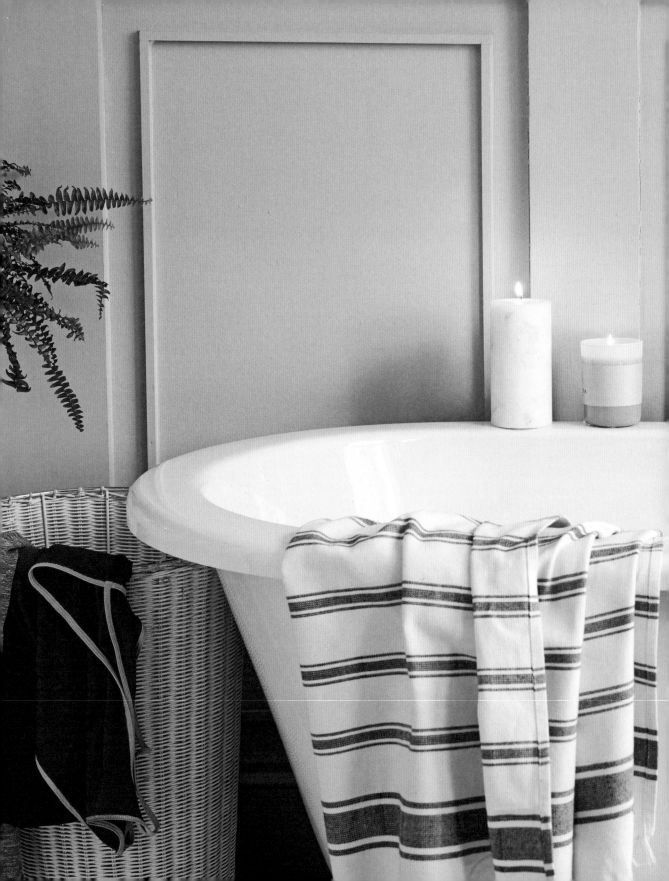

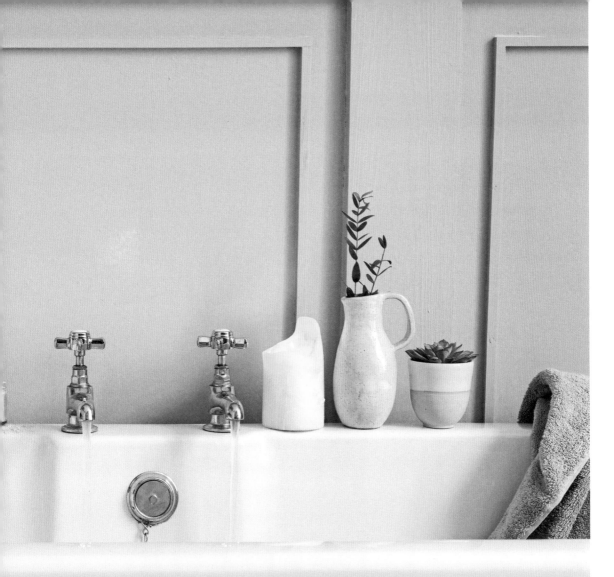

Mindset

"

STRONG ENOUGH TO STAND ALONE, SMART ENOUGH TO KNOW WHEN YOU NEED HELP AND BRAVE ENOUGH TO ASK FOR IT.

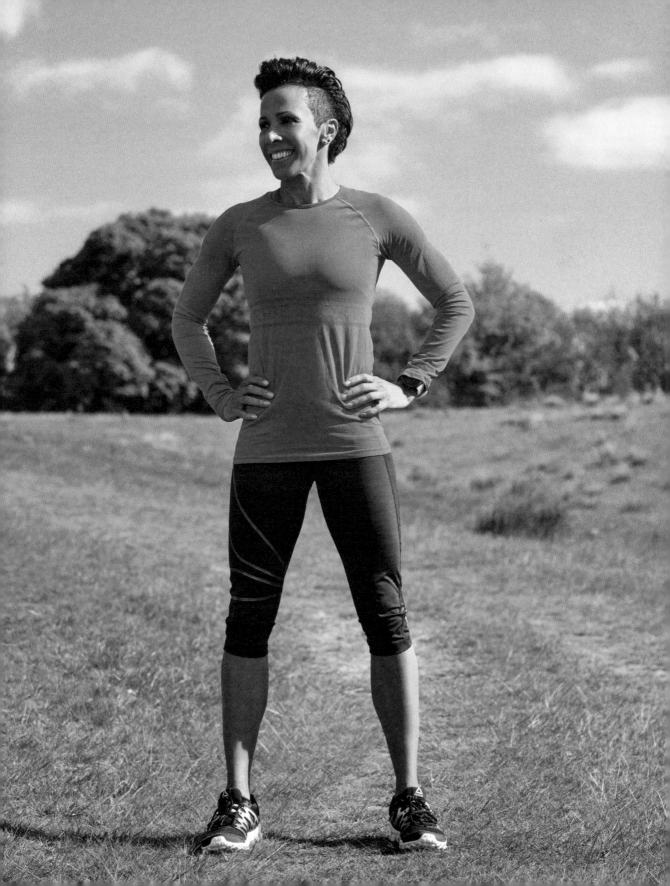

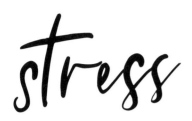

stress

Mindset is so important to a healthy lifestyle and I have tried to identify the many ways the mind can function and how how it affects us. Our mood impacts on everything – the key is to recognise that we can help ourselves by looking after ourselves and our minds.

We can all reach points in our lives where we feel overwhelmed. It's part of being human and the life events that impact our sense of wellbeing are often unavoidable. Difficult situations happen and we may feel we have no choice in how things play out (for example, loss and endings, illness or injury). However, we can choose how we respond to the situation even when painful feelings are inevitably involved. Giving ourselves time to recover from an overwhelming period in our life is key on the road to recovery.

STRESS & YOU

Stress is a human response when our body perceives danger. We will all experience feelings of stress at times in our lives and in many ways it is a very natural reaction that our bodies need to function, so not all stress is negative. A low level of stress can sometimes be a good thing as it can motivate us to get things done and meet targets (some people describe how they thrive on stress) but when it becomes overwhelming it can start to cause problems.

- An emotional and/or physical reaction to being under pressure
- Feeling overwhelmed from taking on too much
- Overthinking a particular worry
- A situation that feels out of our control
- Facing big changes in life
- Multiple responsibilities
- Periods of uncertainty

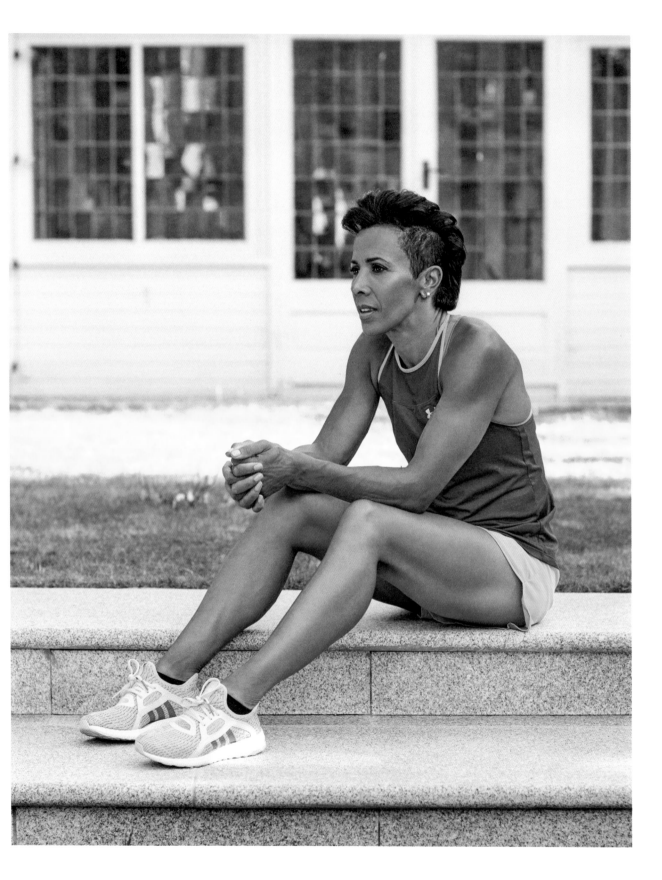

Most of us are familiar with feelings of stress and these feelings usually occur when there is an imbalance in our life. We can get a sense of feeling flooded by difficult thoughts, emotions and physical sensations and we can start to feel like things have got out of control.

There can be many reasons for feeling stressed. We may be facing one big event or it could be a build up of multiple smaller issues. If we find ourselves saying things like 'I'm stressed out' or 'This is so stressful' we may be describing a situation such as the following:

When it becomes overwhelming, too much stress can start to cause problems

SIGNS OF STRESS

Sometimes we find it a bit harder to name stress and we don't always realise that it is stress that we are suffering from. It is likely that we may feel some of the following:

- Impatience
- Nervousness
- Fearful
- Isolated
- Distracted
- Depressed
- Overthinking, overwhelmed and finding it difficult to 'switch off'
- Tension that stops you from enjoying yourself or having fun
- Angry (both internally and externally)

Stress can also manifest itself through physical sensations, including some of the following:

- Feeling physically tense in your body
- Tightness and aches in your muscles
- Tension in your face i.e. frowning or tightening your lower jaw
- Shallow breathing
- Tired eyes
- A 'wired' sensation in your body
- Tiredness but difficulty sleeping
- Loss of libido
- Problems with your digestive system
- Tension headaches or dizziness

As well as what we are feeling emotionally and physically, there are some telltale signs of stress in our behaviour too:

- Avoiding getting things done and then worrying about missing deadlines
- Avoiding certain situations and people
- Worrying about small things and things that may never happen
- Being irritable and angry towards others
- Being indecisive and finding it difficult to concentrate
- Biting your nails and picking your skin
- Restlessness
- Feeling tearful and fragile
- Being excessively early or late

It is important to highlight that we are all different and therefore react differently in certain situations. What stresses one person out to the point of sleepless nights and overthinking, can trigger much less of a reaction in another person. It is important not to fall into the trap of comparing yourself to others when looking at these reactions.

It often doesn't matter how stressful a situation actually is – it's how we perceive and react to it that's important. This can be because of your past experiences, your current level of self-esteem or whether you usually interpret things positively or negatively. Other factors that determine how stressed you feel can be whether you have experienced a particular life event before, feeling shocked by a life event, the amount of other pressures you are facing (financial, family, relationships) and also the amount of support you have available to you.

my story

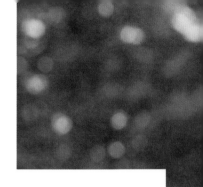

'I WILL NEVER GET OVER LOSING MY MOTHER, I WILL JUST HAVE TO LEARN TO LIVE WITH IT.'

My mum, who I affectionately called 'Mother Dear', had multiple myeloma, a cancer that forms in a type of white blood cell called a plasma cell. Multiple Myeloma causes cancer cells to accumulate in the bone marrow where they crowd out healthy blood cells. Her passing on 7th August 2017 was, without doubt, the worst day of my life. Although she received great care and treatment to prolong her life, in the end, there were too many complications to save her.

My mum had initially been diagnosed at the end of 2014 and it was an unbelievable shock to her and the rest of us. She went from having lingering backache to broken ribs and, in what seemed like an instant, straight to the devastating diagnosis. It all seemed so surreal, almost as if it was happening to someone else. The treatment process that followed was, on one hand, absolute hell for her and, on the other, gave her (and us) the hope we needed. During her initial treatment she suffered quite a lot with depression and also developed diabetes as a result of the steroids. Alongside this she suffered the agony of losing her hair and dealing with sores because of the drugs, shingles and a whole host of other terrible conditions as her immune system was attacked. But she was a fighter and, every time she was given a new drug, she saw it as a new lease of life.

She died on a Monday and I wasn't there. I was out of the country on a pre-planned trip, after spending nearly every day with her the previous week, visiting her in hospital and keeping her company during various treatments. I spent a lot of time with mum to keep her company as there's nothing worse than being somewhere you don't want to be be on your own. But Mother Dear wanted things her way – she hated being in hospital (as we all do) and she was desperate to get back to her own bed and so, after speaking to my family on the Friday before, I took her home. Not one of us expected what would happen over the next three days.

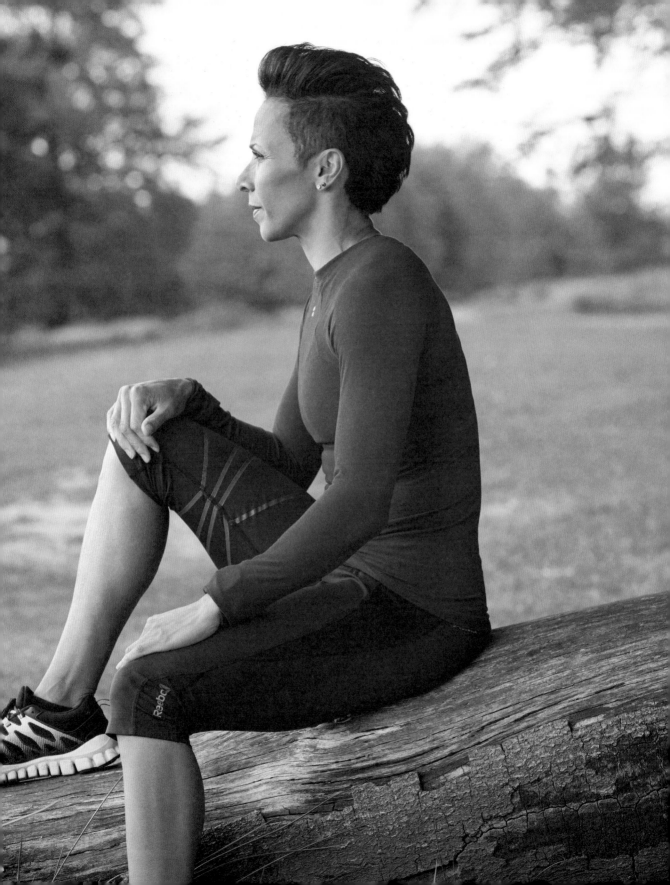

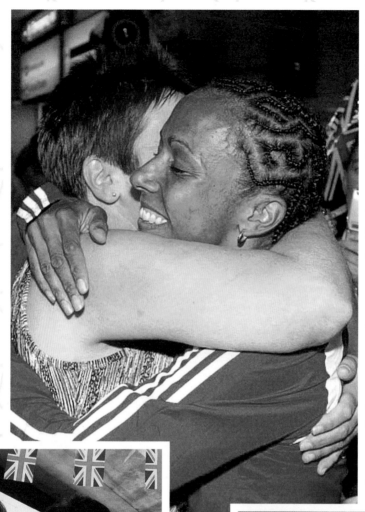

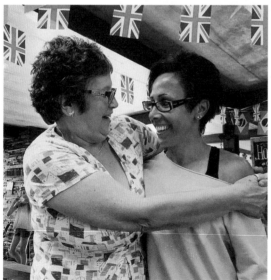

I will hold on to the fact
she was proud of me.

I could go into all the detail here, but it is still all too raw for me. I was far away from everyone and, out of the blue, one of my brothers sent me a text on the Monday morning saying that Mother Dear was not in a good way. What happened in the next 20 minutes changed my life forever.

I locked myself in the toilet of the hotel where I was staying, got some scissors and cut my leg – all I wanted to do was 'take the pain away' from my mum. I knew it was wrong as soon as I did it and that it wouldn't help. At that point, the phone went again and I rushed to get it. Mum passed away 10 minutes later.

The next 12 hours were an utter blur and I can hardly remember anything except an extended plane and boat journey home. The friend I was with organised the whole journey back and one of my best friends picked us up from the airport to take me to the hospital so I could see Mum.

I was numb and, as I write this, I still am. Part of my deep anguish is that I was not there with her the morning that she died. Another thing that really breaks me is that I know she really did not want to die – just a couple of weeks before she did, she was crying as she told me that she was too young to go and that conversation will stay with me forever.

I still well up and get emotional for different reasons, part of me wonders if that will ever stop. I see something my mum would have liked in the shops – but she's not there to get it for, I go somewhere she wanted to go – but she's not there to come. I get given a goodie bag and remember that she always had to look through it first – but she's not there give it to.

I was considering counselling as I know a lot of people benefit from talking to an independent person about their troubles, but I wanted to get the first anniversary out the way, as it was a huge milestone. I did not cope well with it. I felt like I was having a mini breakdown but instead of totally retreating I poured my heart out to thousands of people on social media. Why? Because it helped to talk through the process and be real. In all honesty, it helped me and I wanted to help others through my pain.

What happened has made me realise that life is not a guarantee, it's a privilege, we need to cherish what we do and have, but also remember to live our lives to the full. Getting stuck into my fitness and, I hope, inspiring and motivating others to be the best version of themselves is the perfect way to get lost in the moment and forget my own worries – seeing people smile makes me smile.

How to deal with stress

The good news is that there are various steps you can take to help you manage feelings of stress. Again, different things work for different people, so if one exercise or approach doesn't seem to help much, be open to trying something else.

how to cope:

It is important to know that when we are overwhelmed, there are small things that we can do to take back some control. I believe that consistently thinking positively, eating well and moving are keys to overall balance and happiness. However, when stress threatens to overwhelm us, it can be hard to see a clear way forward. But remember, your mind holds all the power. The decision to either give up and let stress drown you, or take a deep breath and achieve some small steps to put yourself back in the driving seat, is yours alone.

We dedicate so much time to training our bodies, we forget about dedicating some energy to our minds. Learn to celebrate the small things you have achieved and, once you have mastered this, you will be unstoppable! Life is about being emotionally fit and healthy as well as what you put on your plate and how you pass your time in the gym.

It is hard to avoid stress, but constant elevated stress levels increase the release of cortisol, which in turn increases blood sugar levels. Other studies have shown that it can also be linked to high blood pressure. It is important to control how we react to stress if we can. Here are some tips that work for me.

TIPS FOR MANAGING STRESS AND KEEPING YOUR MIND HAPPY:

1. **TRY AND DO ONE POSITIVE THING EVERY DAY AND WRITE IT DOWN** – It will help to finish the day by looking at what you have achieved.

2. **UNDERSTAND SITUATIONS THAT EXACERBATE YOUR FEELINGS OF ANXIETY** – For example, journal how you feel and discuss any feelings of anxiety with your support network.

3. **TRY TO FIT IN SOME KIND OF EXERCISE THAT YOU ENJOY** – It enables you to switch off your mind if it is racing, which can also help with sleep as mind and body are closely linked.

4. **WE ACHIEVE WHAT WE BELIEVE WE CAN** – So write down some short- medium- and long-term goals to help you keep focused. Everything I have ever achieved is because I think anything is possible with enough dedication and hard work. Our thoughts set the standard for what we make happen and having goals provides great focus.

5. **STOP COMPARING YOURSELF TO OTHERS** – and remember everyone is different with their own hopes and goals. Concentrate on yourself and don't look over your shoulder at others.

6. **BE REALISTIC AND DON'T GIVE UP** – For example, if you have a bad food day, miss a training session or allow the fear to swamp you, it's okay. Just start again the following day. Setbacks and disappointments are part of life.

7. **DELEGATE AND ASK FOR HELP WHEN YOU NEED IT** – It's okay if you can't do everything yourself. Asking for some advice will often take the stress out of the situation.

SLEEP

Sleep is one of the most overlooked and undervalued aspects of life, both in its quantity and quality. Many studies have shown that lack of good sleep (or any sleep at all) increases stress levels, decreases energy levels and appetite and, generally, makes everything feel much worse than it might actually be. It also affects how well we exercise and how our muscles repair themselves. Getting good-quality sleep (and enough of it) is vital if we are to try to have a calmer and more productive mind. Things that can help, include:

- If you are stressed about how much you have to do, make a list before bed. Planning the next day with things listed in order of priority is a great way to clear your mind before going to sleep.

- Turn off your devices! (I am so bad at this!) Everything is the touch of a button away and we often have everything on our phone, including work emails, social media and depressing world news. We can feel worse by scrolling through the social media accounts of others, often unhelpfully comparing ourselves (and our lives) to ones edited for show. Try to turn off your phone at least one hour before you want to go to sleep. Invest in an alarm clock and leave your phone in another room, away from temptation.

- Have a routine so that your body recognises when it is time to prepare for sleep. Run a bath and read a book, whatever you do should be relaxing and not involve a screen!

WHAT PRESSES YOUR 'STRESS BUTTON'?

Figuring out what presses your stress button can help you to notice the signs of stress earlier and so help to make a plan to try a different way forward. Often it is not possible to avoid stressful situations or, indeed some of the triggers of stress, but taking time to work out what contributes towards your own triggers can help you to understand why you get stressed.

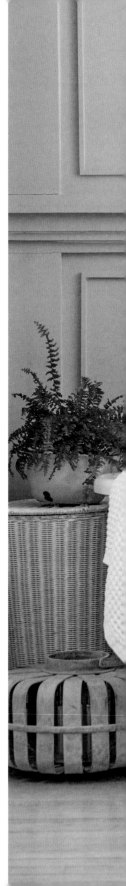

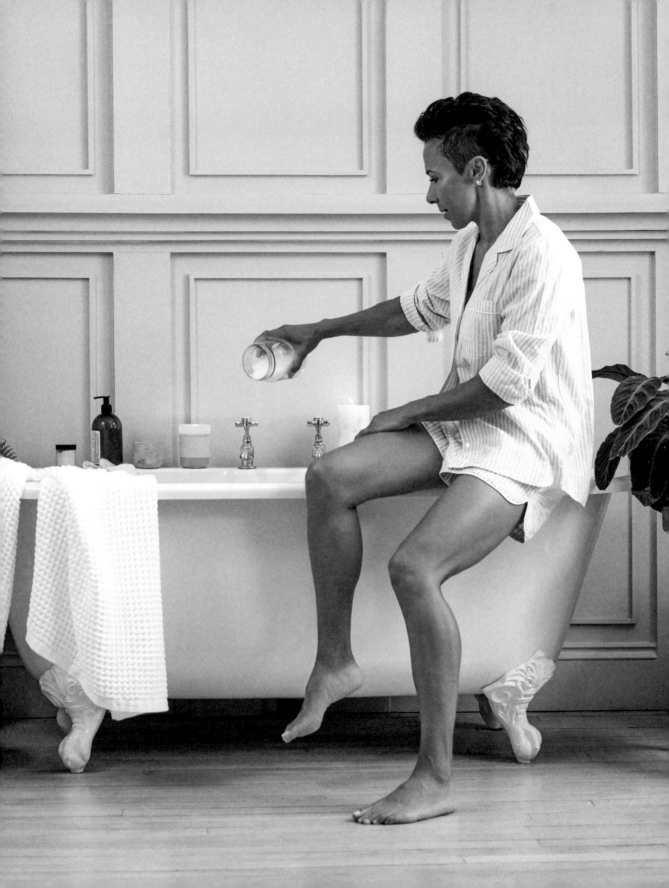

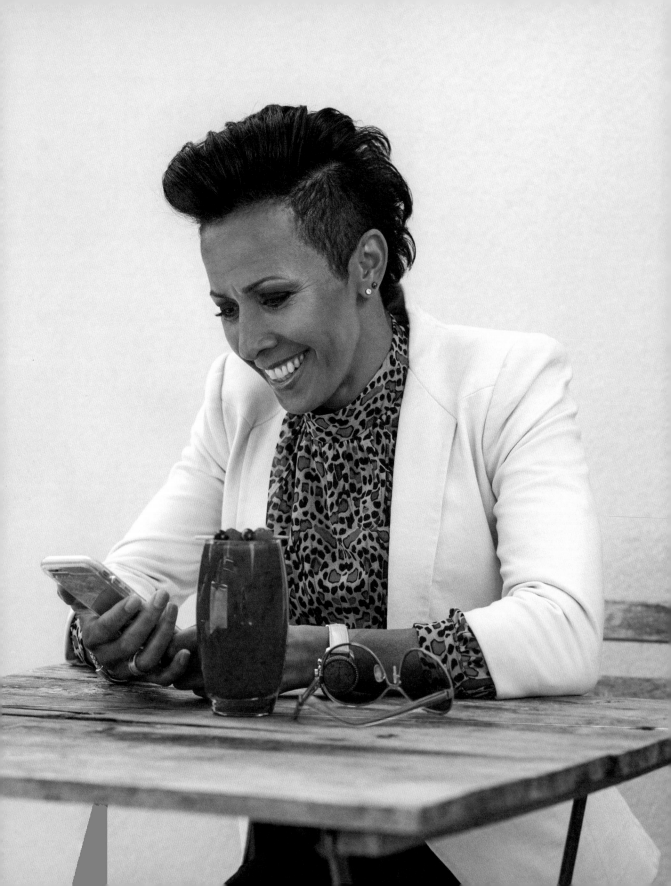

TIME MANAGEMENT

When I was in the military, I had no problem at all with time management – being on time was non-negotiable. When I was racing, there were also timelines for competing. The race wouldn't wait for you if you were late, so everything from what time you left home, warmed up, right through to the start time, had to be planned ahead.

However, these days, I am not the best at managing my time for the following reasons:

- Too much going on and rushing from one thing to the other.

- Cramming too much into one day.

- Juggling my various commitments, especially as they need different things from me: fitness, motivational speaking, emails, social media and being a café owner.

- Unforeseen circumstances, normally due to the amount of travel I do, for example, delayed trains or flights.

```
THINGS I COULD DO BETTER TO AVOID STRESS

1. Plan ahead more
2. Get everything ready the day/night before
3. Don't cram so much into a day
4. Don't take on too much
```

How you manage your time and organise your daily routines can impact how stressed you feel. Making some changes can help you to feel that you are taking control of your day-to-day life and how you spend your time.

SETTING GOALS

Being in sport is great for setting goals and targets. As soon as I decided to run the London Marathon in 2016, I had the exact date in my diary to plan for. I then worked out how many weeks I had in order to be at my best for that date. Once I had done that, I looked at a couple of training plans that I thought I could fit into my hectic lifestyle alongside work and family commitments, fundraising events, travelling for speaking engagements, etc. I then set the overall time goal I hoped to achieve, which allowed me to set shorter milestones like what pace I wanted do a certain run in, how many rest days I would have and how much I would increase my distance by each weekend in order to be confident I could run my best race.

When you feel stressed, it's tempting to set yourself big targets in order to try to bring about big change. This can often create a situation where more pressure is piled on to reach these targets and then disappointment when they are not met. When setting targets, consider what balance you have in your life. It's important to have a variety of activities and things that are both good for you and that interest you. We all have to deal with everyday mundane tasks as well as some tasks that are stressful. Mixing these in with things that you enjoy will help you to feel more balanced.

BALANCE

I believe in balance, whether it's with my current fitness regime, food intake, going out or relaxing. In terms of fitness, I enjoy a mix of sessions and body part specific training. When I'm trying to focus on maintaining my fitness I do this by running, cycling, weight training, HIIT and circuit training – this gives me a good variety of cardio, strength and endurance training.

When it comes to my food I don't like the word diet, I prefer to use food intake. Despite all sorts of myths and theories about weight, everyone should know that it's all about what you consume. Fitness and how many calories you burn also have a huge impact on this equation, but, as the saying goes, you can't out-train a bad diet.

I really enjoy my food. I particularly like sweets, chocolate, Indian takeaways and Thai food and I don't deprive myself of these but I don't eat them every day. Luckily, I also feel good when I'm eating fruit and veg and I know that proteins like fish, chicken, pulses are good for me so I make sure I have variety in a day.

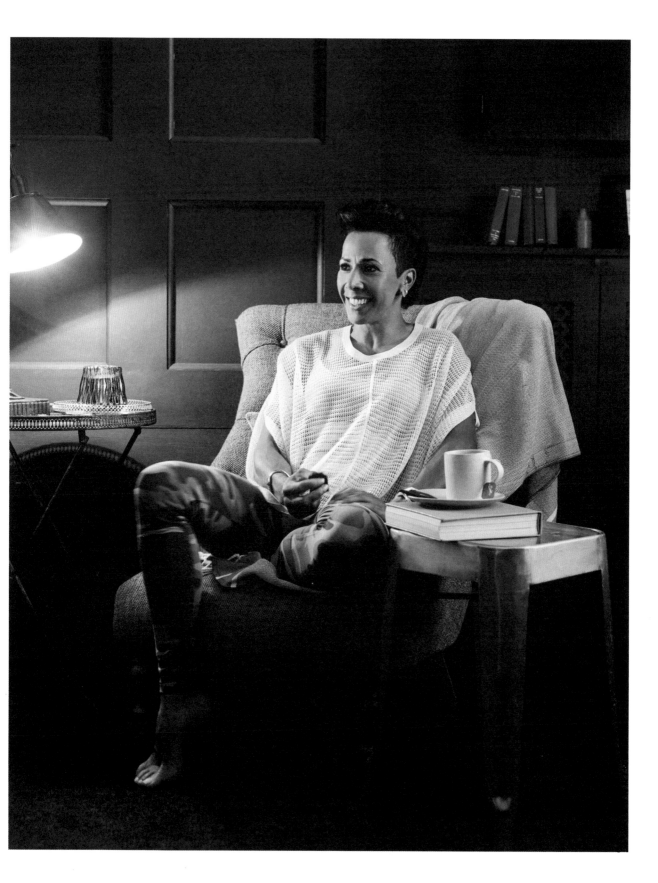

WHEN DOES YOUR STRESS BUTTON
GET PRESSED?

In order to gauge your level of stress, it can be helpful to practise putting a number on your stress levels, so you can stay in tune with the physical, emotional and behavioural effects when your stress button is being pressed. For me, the below list can be triggers for feelings of stress and being overwhelmed:

- Being overtired
- Feeling of being let down
- Not sure of the direction I am going, either in work or my personal life
- Death

To start to get to know your own stress levels, check where you are on this gauge in different situations. For example, you might notice the sensation of a small amount of stress either physically or emotionally and say to yourself, 'I'm feeling around a 3–4'. At another time, for example, before an important meeting, or if you are running late for an appointment, you will notice your stress levels rising and you might feel around an 6.

This exercise is easy once you start to practise it and once you notice what number your stress level is at, you can take a moment to consider how you might be able to bring the level down to a lower number.

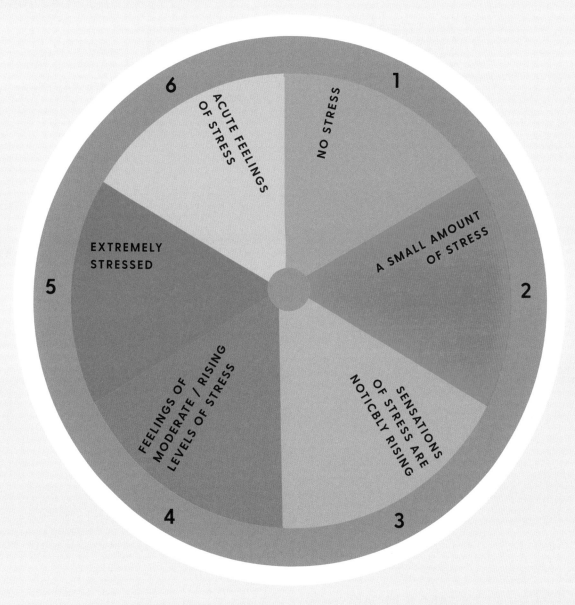

6 ACUTE FEELINGS OF STRESS

1 NO STRESS

2 A SMALL AMOUNT OF STRESS

5 EXTREMELY STRESSED

3 SENSATIONS OF STRESS ARE NOTICBLY RISING

4 FEELINGS OF MODERATE / RISING LEVELS OF STRESS

Here are some practical ways in which you can start to change some of your triggers and lower the stress level number:

>> **ARE YOU A MORNING OR EVENING PERSON?**
I have a slight problem being both a morning and an evening person because of my sleep pattern and that probably contributes to some of my stress. So I have started to use relaxation techniques and not go to bed so close to exercising.

Identifying which time of the day you have the most energy and focus and pre-planning important tasks for those times may help with successful outcomes.

>> **LEARN TO SAY 'NO'**
Taking on too much at once can cause and/or contribute towards feeling overwhelmed and stressed. Some people have difficulty in saying no to requests and before you know it, you have said yes to so many people, you no longer have time for yourself and it becomes very difficult to do any one task well. This can make you feel more under pressure.

I get asked to do so many things, such as support numerous charities, and in the past I have felt really bad saying no, as if I was letting people down. Now I ensure that I have easier ways to support and communicate with charities, even if it can't be in person, like sending signed autograph cards and videos. I also make sure that each year I decide on which charities I will support as well as my own Dame Kelly Holmes Trust, so that I stick to giving them my full attention instead of spreading myself thin.

>> **LISTS, LISTS, LISTS**
Making lists of things that you have to do, and arranging them in order of importance, can help you to focus on getting back in control and successfully achieving tasks. There is also something very satisfying about ticking an item off the list once it is complete. Some people find making a timetable helpful, to help with managing time more effectively. This can be work-related tasks, home life, or both.

>> **TAKE A BREAK**
While ticking off the tasks on your to-do list, ensure you leave time to take breaks. Try not to rush through tasks. Take things more slowly to invite a calmer approach to getting things done. Over time, this will help you to build your concentration and, in turn, be more productive.

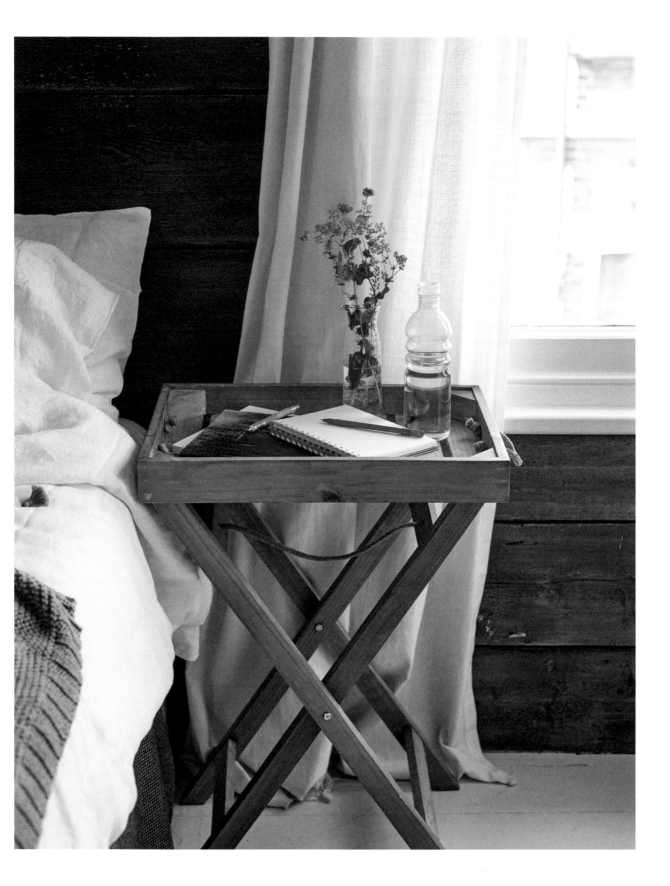

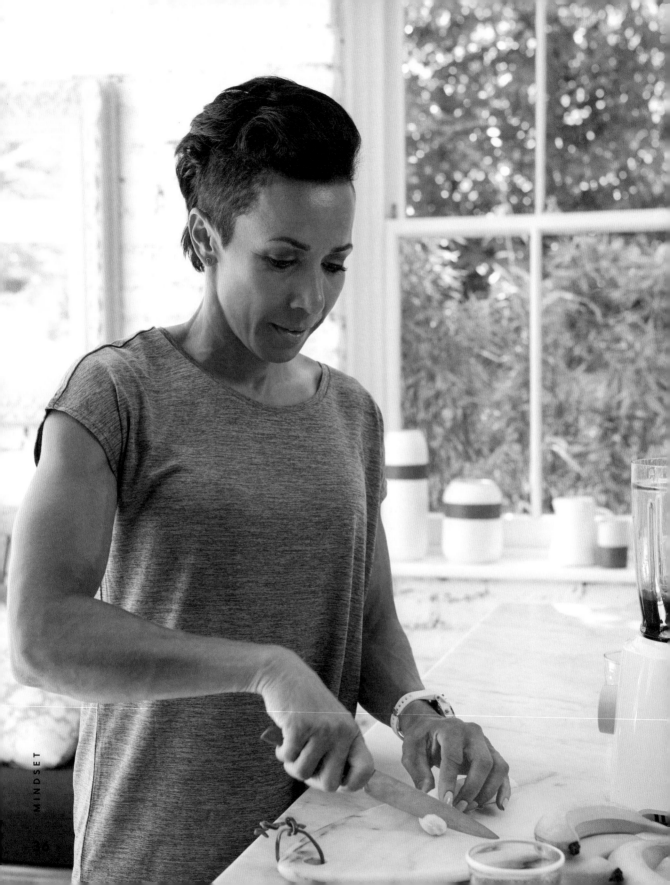

A strong sense of wellbeing and resilience will not only help your ability to recover from setbacks, but also help you to be more able to deal with change.

>> **ASK FOR HELP**

Don't be afraid to delegate tasks that need to be done. It is important to manage your expectations of other people either agreeing and/or carrying out tasks in the same way that you do. Letting go of these expectations can help with any feelings of 'I have to do it all'.

>> **YOUR PHYSICAL HEALTH**

Looking after your physical health can dramatically improve mental wellbeing and help to reduce feelings of stress. Make it a priority to get enough sleep, be physically active and understand your eating patterns to make better, healthier choices. All of these will help you to feel good about yourself physically, mentally and emotionally.

>> **ACCEPTING THE THINGS THAT YOU CANNOT CHANGE**

It can be very empowering to reach the point of accepting the things that we cannot control or change. Redirecting your focus to things in your life where you do have control will help you to feel more in charge of your choices and result in you being more productive and focused.

>> **BUILDING EMOTIONAL RESILIENCE**

A great sense of wellbeing and resilience will not only help your ability to recover from setbacks, but also help you to be more able to deal with change, even when it is unexpected and uncomfortable. Emotional resilience is a skill that anyone can take steps to practise and learn.

Resilience can help you in a number of difficult situations including experiencing any kind of loss such as losing your job, the break-up of a significant relationship or friendship, dealing with difficult individuals both at work and in your personal life, being the victim of crime or injustice or any of the stressful scenarios listed in this section.

GETTING TO KNOW YOUR REACTIONS

You can start to understand your own level of resilience by imagining yourself in a scenario where you have faced a setback and noticing that you are feeling negative emotions. Here is a list of possible unhelpful and helpful reactions. Rate yourself for each of these statements to identify your reactions.

UNHELPFUL REACTIONS WHEN FACING A SETBACK

1. I isolate myself from others.
2. I avoid uncomfortable situations and try to avoid negative feelings.
3. I start to recall other things in my life that have gone wrong.
4. I regularly drink alcohol or use drugs to make me feel better for a while, even though I know they are harmful to me.
5. I think of myself as a victim of the situation.
6. I suppress my feelings.
7. I reach for something to eat in between usual mealtimes.

When I am starting to get stressed I sometimes have to do what I call 'flicking the switch'. I can get so wrapped up in things that are on my mind that I start being consumed by them. Like when I have fallen out with someone in my personal life and feel frustrated, hurt or let down it takes over my brain and I get stressed and anxious.

Now I try these helpful reactions and find they work. The easier ones for me are numbers 2, 3 and 4.

1. I notice my thoughts but don't get caught up in overthinking.
2. I talk to someone that I trust about how I am feeling.
3. I go to the gym or find some other way of exercising.
4. I try new ways of calming myself down such as meditation, relaxation or breathing exercises.
5. I pause, start to figure out a solution and take a first step.
6. I recall times when I have successfully dealt with problems in the past.
7. I record how I'm feeling in my diary.

Talking about your feelings is a sign of personal strength and of being able to take control of your life. It can be difficult to know how to start a conversation about your feelings or worries, but some of the tips below might help you to manage the process:

- Find the right moment for the conversation – you want to have time to talk and not be interrupted.

- You might find it easier to start the conversation when you are doing something else – you're out for a walk or travelling in the car together.

- Knowing what to say always feels hard.

- It's okay to start off by saying you have been going through a tough time and to describe what you've been thinking and feeling.

- It is normal to feel nervous. You might worry about how people will react, but when you let someone know you need their help, they will usually respond positively.

WHO DO I TALK TO ABOUT STRESS?

Talk to someone you trust such as your partner, a family member, a friend or a colleague. People will listen and give you support if you let them know how you're feeling. It might also help the people you care about – if you open up about your feelings, they might do the same. Even being in other people's company can be beneficial. If you find it too difficult then also consider talking to a GP or counsellor.

TREATMENT FOR STRESS

If you are struggling with stress, and require additional help there are treatments available. It is advisable to talk to your GP in the first instance. Aside from meditation, your doctor may suggest one of the following: talking therapies with a trained professional,including counselling, psychotherapy and Cognitive Behavioral Therapy; exercise; complimentary and alternative therapies, which may include yoga, meditation, acupuncture, aromatherapy, reflexology and massage; attending a mindfulness course or stretching. Regularly stretching has been shown to reduce mental tension and, when combined with mindful breathing techniques, may also help to decrease anxiety and depression.

PTSD AND HOW YOU CAN RECOGNISE IT . . .

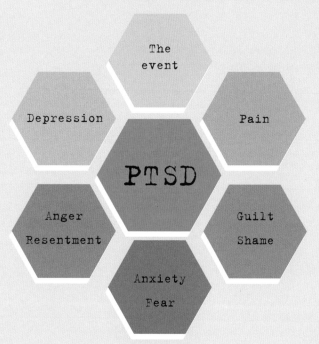

There is a moment for some when it becomes clear they are suffering from something more extreme than everyday stress and depression. Something that could have been triggered by a life-altering event or situation that has left them deeply scarred. Although this term can be used for the victims of multiple situations (including sexual crimes), having been in the army, I have seen many scenarios that could fall into the category of post-traumatic stress disorder (PTSD). PTSD is a mental disorder that can develop after a person is exposed to a traumatic event, such as sexual assault, warfare, traffic collisions, or other threat on their life. It is vital for those affected to get the help they need. If not, the repercussions can last a lifetime and have an effect long after the horror of their war (whatever that is for them) is over.

Meditation and mindfulness are fantastic (non-medical) ways of overcoming trauma and stress. It isn't just about reciting your favourite mantras, it is about focusing on what you are doing in the present moment, rather than being overwhelmed and letting it pass you by. It is about paying attention to your own thoughts and internal dialogue, and accepting them. It's about feeling and the world around you. A clearer sense of awareness can also help us spot worrying signs of stress and upset at an earlier stage, meaning we are sometimes lucky enough (like Natalie opposite) to catch them before they escalate.

Natalie's story

Natalie, an investment banker working in the city, went to a mindful meditation workshop four years ago. She was struggling with work-related stress and not being able to switch off from her busy mind. She was smoking heavily, unable to sleep at night and had started to lose her hair, which she had to have cut very short because of the bald patches that were appearing. Natalie wasn't convinced that meditation would help and to begin with found it almost impossible to sit still for the guided meditation exercise. Her brain continued to race with thoughts and she had a constant urge to fidget. Natalie did, however, like 'the idea' of the core concepts of mindfulness and even when it was a challenge, established a regular practice for herself.

It's been a journey over several years, but Natalie has made some very important choices. Here's how she describes the changes she has experienced:

case studies

'To begin with I found it very, very hard to relax and to stop the thoughts racing round and round my head. I practised short breathing exercises, three or four times per day to being with. A bit like going on a run, the more I practised, the further I found I was able to go with my mindfulness meditation practice.*

It is not a quick fix but more of a lifestyle change. It takes time. Just in the same way that you wouldn't be able to run a marathon without some dedicated practice.

So four years on, I feel in a calmer place. I have the same career but I am much less stressed. I do wonderful meditation exercises lasting 15–20 minutes on a busy commuter train, without anyone else knowing I am doing it! It sets me up for the day and calms me down on the way home. I take walks in the city at lunchtime, I run and I practise yoga.

I am so glad that I chose to make these changes and that I stuck with this new lifestyle. I have stopped smoking altogether and my hair has now grown back and reaches my shoulders again.'

Fall down seven times, get up eight

I LOVE THIS JAPANESE SAYING

There isn't enough space here to adequately address Japanese culture and ways of thinking, but this Japanese proverb reflects an important and shared ideal: '*Nana korobi ya oki*' (literally: seven falls, eight getting up), which means fall down seven times and get up eight. This speaks to the Japanese concept of resilience. No matter how many times you get knocked down, you get up again. Even if you should fall one thousand times, you just keep getting up and trying again. You can see this ethic reinforced in all facets of Japanese culture including education, business, sports, martial arts, the Zen arts, etc. It is especially important to remember the sentiment expressed in this proverb when times are dark. There are no quick fixes in life and anything of real worth will necessarily take much struggle and perseverance. Success does not have to be fast — what's more important is that you simply do your absolute best and remain persistent. I use this analogy in relation to my athletics career when I talk about being knocked down for seven years (because of injury) and standing up in the eighth year to win double Olympic gold.

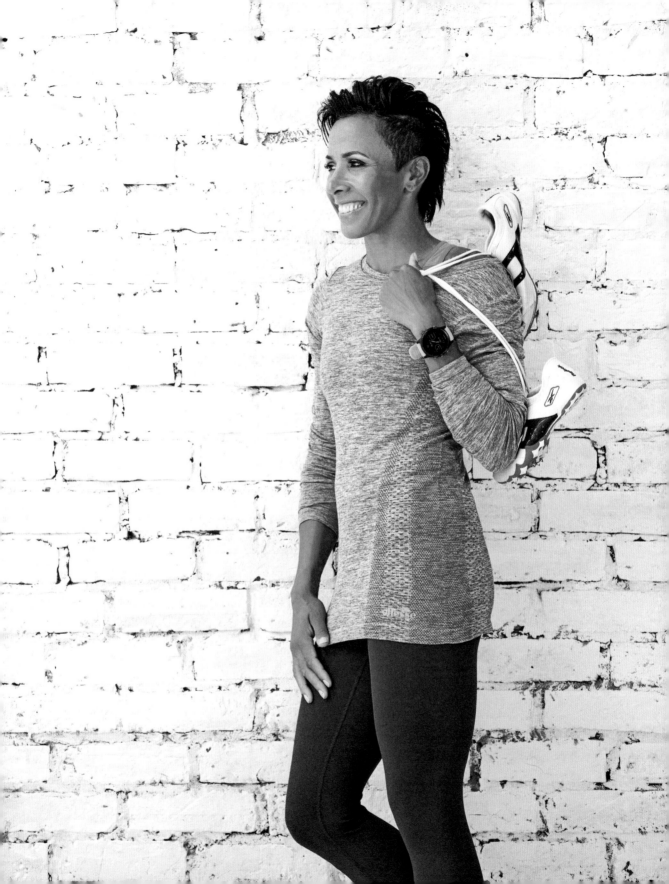

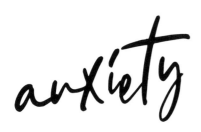

anxiety

Anxiety is another way of describing a sense of fear and nervousness. Sometimes rational, sometimes irrational but always uncomfortable. Similar to stress, feeling anxious usually comes hand in hand with feeling a loss of control.

Feelings of anxiety can occur when we are worried about things that are happening in our lives, things that haven't happened yet or things that may never happen at all (i.e. thoughts that begin with 'what if...?').

Anxiety is a natural way to feel fear as part of a human survival mechanism. Without these feelings we would take far too many risks and without the fear mechanism kicking in, we would most certainly face dangerous consequences through not taking enough care. A life without any sense of fear would be an unsafe place to be.

Many people are affected by feelings of anxiety that are not helpful. This is most commonly when our anxious reactions to thoughts and situations become completely out of proportion with the situation we are faced with.

I felt most anxious during my athletics career because of having very specific goals that had a lot of variables – no matter how I prepared or what I did, there was no guarantee I would win and this anxiety around potential failure definitely led to the start of my self-harming.

Setting up my charity in 2008 was hugely stressful and made me anxious – mainly due to how some people within the various organisations treated me. There were definitely those who were there more for an ego trip and less for doing good. Have you had a situation when you felt bullied and intimidated by others? It's a horrible feeling.

My charity has been going for over 10 years now because I realised that, whilst things were upsetting me, I believed in what I was trying to achieve and was not going to let people put me down. It was hard but it was an example of when sometimes we have to take control even though we don't actually have any. I also had to adopt similar methods around the time of my mother's death because, suddenly, I had no control of the outcome.

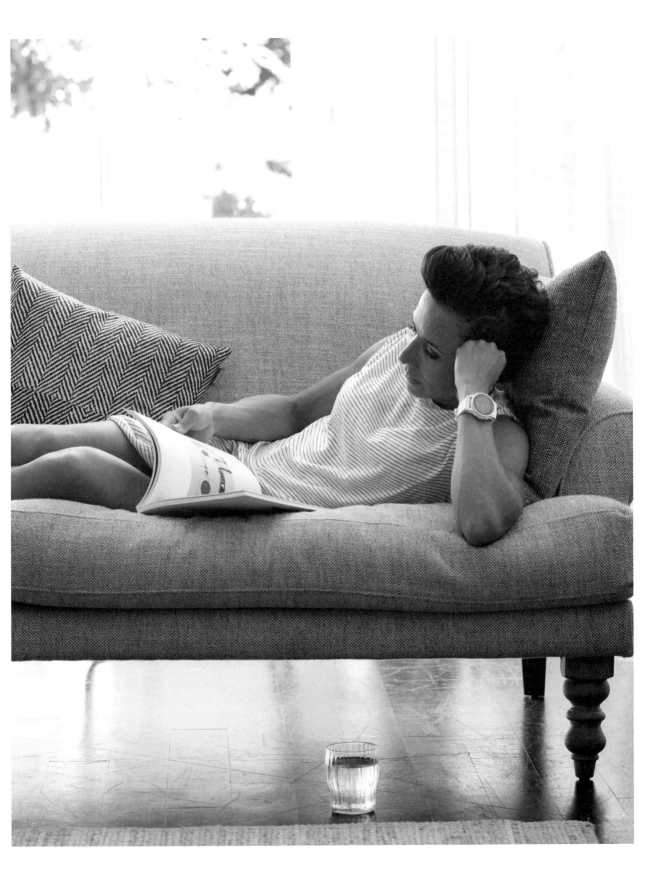

SIGNS OF ANXIETY

ANXIETY CAN OFTEN HAVE A PHYSICAL IMPACT ON OUR BODY. HERE ARE SOME OF THE PHYSICAL SENSATIONS AND SYMPTOMS ASSOCIATED WITH ANXIETY:

- A sense of restlessness
- 'Butterflies' or a churning feeling in your stomach, feeling sick
- Blushing
- Difficulty sleeping
- Panic attacks
- Dizziness
- Aches and pains
- Shallow, quicker breathing
- A sense of disconnection with yourself or the world around you

---

WHEN WE ARE SUFFERING FROM ANXIETY, IT IS LIKELY THAT WE MAY THINK AND FEEL SOME OF THE FOLLOWING:

- Nervousness and a feeling of fear
- Worrying and afraid of the 'worst-case scenario' happening
- Tense and unable to relax
- Self-conscious
- Fear that a panic attack might happen
- Concerned about what other people think, assuming others are annoyed or upset with you
- Overthinking a situation with it going over and over in your head

I once went on a TV programme called *Mission Survive* with Bear Grylls, a British adventurer, and seven other people in the public eye. Before the show I thought it best to mention that I had a fear of water and jumping into water from heights, as well as a deep fear of drowning.

As the show progressed, all of my fears seemed to be realised. Every day we came across water as we travelled down through the Costa Rican jungle to the coast over a 12-day period.

Our first task was to jump into what can only be described as a swamp, as our helicopter hovered over it. From a height Bear told us that we must jump and I have never been so petrified in all my life. I actually thought I was going to be physically sick and that, if I jumped, I may not survive. That in itself was debilitating and created so much worry and fear as I imagined the worst-case scenario and I also worried what people would think of me if I didn't do it. Most of all, I was afraid of letting myself down. Well, I did it, it was awful and I never want to do it again, but I think coming face to face with your fear and doing it anyway helps you to deal with other scenarios in a more reflective way.

My time in *Mission Survive* helped me face some of my fears head on

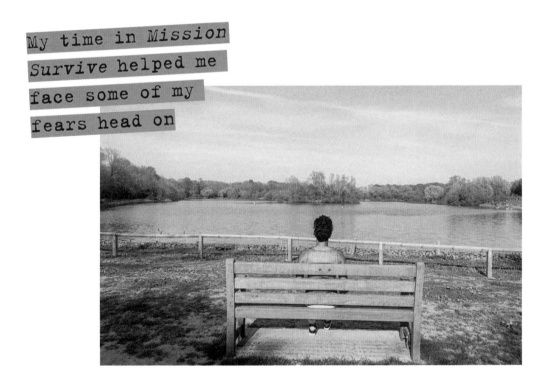

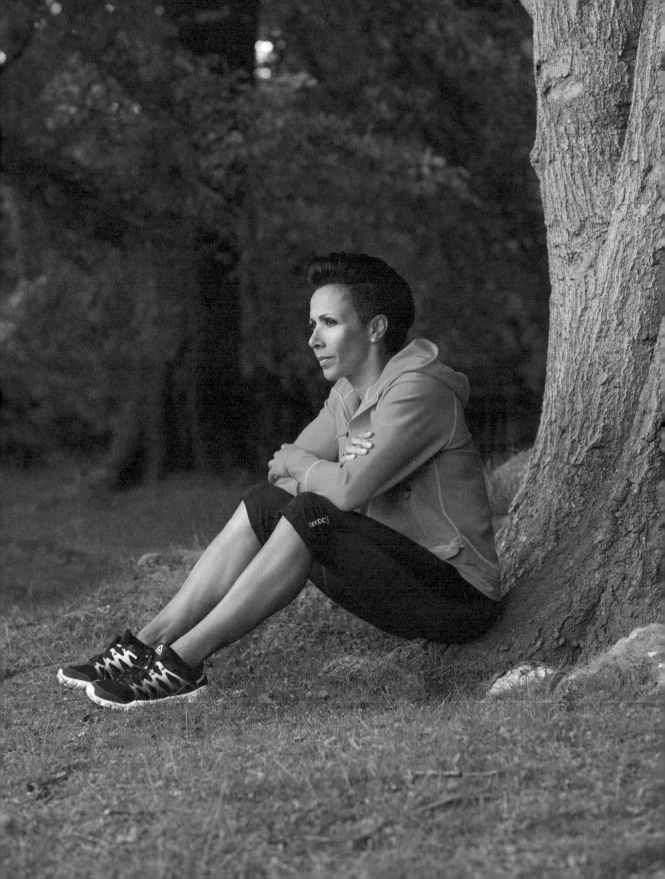

Different types of anxiety

Because we are all individuals, we experience anxiety in lots of different ways and anxious feelings can be triggered by a variety of scenarios. Sometimes we have a general feeling of anxiety and worry about all sorts of different things. Equally, we can experience anxiety around something specific.

Here are some examples of specific types of anxiety:

>> **SOCIAL SITUATIONS** – Fear of situations that include interaction with multiple people, including parties and social gatherings or with colleagues in the workplace. Sometimes referred to 'social anxiety' or dismissed as 'shyness'.

>> **PANIC ATTACKS** – Regularly experiencing a sense of panic or fear at the anticipation of a panic attack happening.

>> **PHOBIAS** – Extreme fear triggered by a particular situation or object.

>> **POST TRAUMA** – Anxiety problems that occur after a traumatic event, which may come in the form of nightmares and flashbacks.

>> **COMPULSIVE (OCD)** – Anxious feelings associated with repeating patterns of behaviour, repetitive thoughts or urges.

>> **HEALTH** – Experiencing anxious thoughts relating to health and illnesses for which there is excessive researching and checking of symptoms.

>> **BODY IMAGE** – Anxiety around your physical appearance and body.

>> **PREGNANCY** – Some new mothers develop anxiety during pregnancy and/or during the post-natal period.

It is advisable that you speak to your GP if you experience any of the above in an extreme way.

Anxiety affecting daily life

Anxiety can affect your daily life choices in a number of ways. This is down to the fearful thoughts, feelings and physical sensations that underlie anxiety. It is not unusual to have trouble looking after yourself or putting a 'self-care' plan in place. You may also find that your work life is impacted, either feeling that you are struggling to concentrate, or not doing a good job or even having difficulty holding down a job. It can be difficult to form new friendships and/ or relationships, or maintain them, which can lead to feelings of isolation. You may feel reluctant to try new things or find it difficult to enjoy existing hobbies and leisure activities.

CAUSES OF ANXIETY

Sometimes it can be very difficult to make sense of why you feel anxious, especially if you can clearly remember a time in your life when it wasn't that way and things seemed very different.

Starting to understand some of the reasons why you began to feel anxious, may set you on the road to gaining control of the feelings, thoughts and sensations. It is hard to change something if you haven't yet made sense, even in a small way, of where it all began.

1. THE PAST
Experiences in the past, even as far back as childhood, can be a trigger for anxiety, even if it doesn't become obvious to you until later in your life.

Going through difficulties in childhood including stressful or traumatic experiences can have a huge impact on you moving forward in your life, even if you were very young. These could include abusive situations (emotional, physical or sexual abuse), neglect, significant, loss particularly through the death of a parent or close family member, distressing school experience such as being bullied, lack of friendships or being left out.

All of the above experiences can impact how safe and secure you felt as a child and this in turn can be a major contributing factor to anxiety later in life. Equally, during our childhood, an adult family member can model anxiety to us and we learn from them, unconsciously, how to be an anxious person.

We are repeating a family narrative. The heartening part of this dynamic is that whatever has been learned, CAN be unlearned.

2. THE PRESENT

As well as things that might have happened in your past, your current situation may also trigger feelings of anxiety, such as facing present issues and problems.

THESE CAN INCLUDE:

- Financial difficulties
- Loss (bereavement, redundancy, relationship)
- Unemployment
- Family problems
- Exhaustion
- Pressure of study and/or exams
- Housing problems
- Abusive situations in professional or personal life

When my mum was diagnosed with Myeloma, it was a big shock to her and my whole family (see pages 20–23). I think at first we were all very positive, as it seemed to be a process that she would get through and survive. She was told she needed a certain drug to control her bloods and then, once that worked, she would be able to get on with 'normal' life. But as the months passed, it very quickly became apparent that, after one successful cycle, the remaining cycles were becoming less and less effective. There was always a different drug to try but she began suffering from more and more complications, until, finally, her body gave up fighting.

Going through difficulties in childhood including stressful or traumatic experiences can have a huge impact on you moving forward in your life.

How to deal with anxiety

>> **TALKING TO SOMEONE YOU TRUST**

Talking about your feelings can be a relief. This can be to a friend or family member. I was in a pretty bad way when my mum passed away. I felt completely lost, anxious and tearful. My friends were very aware of my fragile state of mind and made a point of calling, texting and visiting me. Over the first nine months this was exactly what I needed: longer chats, lunches or a night out with people I trust and love. Not feeling so alone has definitely made the process easier to deal with.

>> **MANAGING YOUR WORRIES**

Trying to stop worrying about things can be extremely difficult when you struggle with anxiety and these thoughts can sometimes feel out of your control. Try setting aside some specific time to focus on the worries. You can do this as an exercise, so that you give yourself permission to think about your worries for a certain amount of time only.

Alternatively, you could try writing your worries down and keeping them in an allotted place. Some people find it useful to keep these notes in an envelope, or in a jar or container. When I worry about something it is on my mind constantly. I try to think of ways to make things easier for myself and imagine ways of solving the scenario. Is there anything physical, practical or financial I can do to sort out the problem? Sometimes, even if it takes a while, I have to keep telling myself in my head that I don't care and sometimes that helps me switch off and stop obsessing about it.

>> **BREATHING EXERCISES**

Breathing exercises can help you with nervousness, anxiety and rising feelings of panic. Your breath is something that comes everywhere with you and you don't need to do anything special to make it happen, and therefore it provides an excellent focus in times of need.

Simply by focusing your attention on your breath and following it in and then back out again, allowing it to flow smoothly and slowly, can help you to feel more grounded. Try to focus your attention on five breaths at a time. Thinking of your breath as an anchor may also help you.

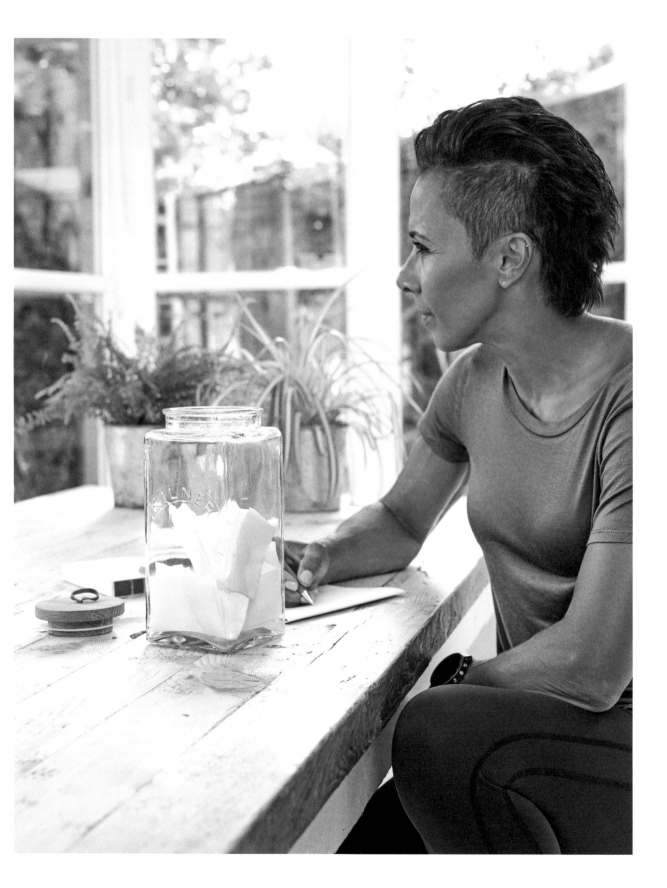

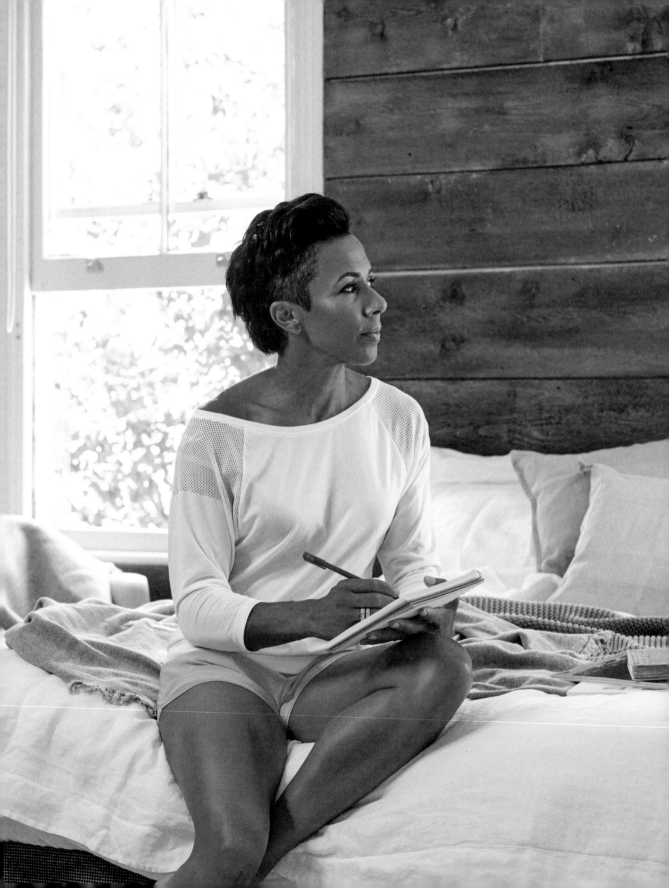

Journalling

Keeping a journal, or diary, might also help. You could start by making some notes on what happens when you get anxious, or start to panic. Over time you might be able to see some patterns emerging and get to know the triggers that start the feelings of anxiety off. You might then start to notice signs of anxiety earlier when the cycle begins to happen. When journalling, it is also important to make a note of the positive things that are happening.

Keeping a journal can be helpful for improving your self-awareness, self-care and mindset, as well as a great way to record your choices, achievements and goals. Here are some suggestions for things to write in your journal:

- RECORDING YOUR THOUGHTS TO EXTERNALISE THEM
  This can help to minimise worries.

- WRITE DOWN YOUR FEELINGS
  as a way of exploring what's going on for you.

- MAP OUT YOUR GOALS
  starting with smaller easier-to-achieve steps.

- RECORD YOUR ACHIEVEMENTS
  to acknowledge what you have done well.

- USE YOUR CREATIVITY AND SKETCH, DOODLE, CREATE
  collages or draw in your journal.

- KEEP A PHOTO DIARY

Remember that your journal does not need to make sense to anyone else but you. It is a place for YOU to express yourself and take note of your own progress.

Alternatively, you could copy the journal template overleaf and complete the sections each day, or each week.

JOURNAL TEMPLATE

DATE..

HOW I AM FEELING TODAY ....

....

TODAY I FEEL GRATEFUL FOR ....

....

CHOICES I MADE TODAY THAT WERE HELPFUL ....

....

THINGS THAT I ACHIEVED TODAY ....

....

SELF-CARE ACTIVITIES ....

MY GOALS ARE ....

....

....

FITNESS GOALS TODAY...

HOURS OF SLEEP LAST NIGHT...

GLASSES OF WATER DRUNK..

TODAY'S NUTRITION NOTES..

Josie's story

In her early 30s Josie found herself struggling with feelings of depression. Josie's depression manifested itself in experiencing anxiety almost every day with a whole range of triggers.

Josie had spoken to her doctor, had tried a number of alternative therapies and was seeing a counsellor. Somehow, whatever she found the energy to try, she seemed to end up feeling worse and overwhelmingly disappointed by 'the next thing' not helping. She started to withdraw more and her anxiety rose because of her feelings of hopelessness.

Despite this, Josie knew that she needed to find a way to start the healing process. During the counselling sessions and conversations with trusted friends, Josie began to revisit and reflect on the difficulties in her childhood. Her father had been absent and her mother an alcoholic. Josie hadn't received the love and nurture that every child is entitled to and needs to help them grow, flourish and be able to express themselves.

During these reflections, Josie started to keep a journal of her thoughts and feelings and, in doing so, soon realised that, in her expressive writing, she had a skill that might help her to understand herself better.

Josie's journal became a record of her journey to self-awareness, a place to safely express how she felt, to write letters to both her parents (that they would never read) to help her process the sadness and anger she felt towards them. She also wrote letters to her younger self, sending kind messages to the lonely eight-year-old Josie, telling her she is loved and she is good enough.

The process of writing this journal was deeply therapeutic for Josie and over time, her journal began to change her mindset. She started to feel more positive and less anxious. In turn, her depression began to lift too. Josie was able to verbalise her feelings through her writing for the first time in her life and in doing so, things became much clearer for her. Ultimately Josie has been able to reach a point of acceptance about her life being different from how she would have liked it to be. This acceptance was the key to Josie finding confidence in herself for the first time in many years.

depression

No matter who you are in life, the job you have and the success that follows, your background, race, colour or physical ability, remember that we are all human.

> Have you ever had moments of doubt, worry, uncertainty, fear, anxiety or stress? *I have too.*
>
> Has it ever gone further than that? Depression, despair, sadness, dejection, misery or feelings of hopelessness? *I have too.*
>
> Or maybe even further, where you have had to 'release' the tension and turn to self-abuse like alcohol, self-harm, drugs or crime? *I have too.*

I have been very open about my depression that led to self-harming, which acted as a release from the deep despair I was feeling. When I first spoke about it in 2005 I don't think people wanted to hear it – they certainly weren't ready for how uncomfortable it made them feel. It was a massive story in the media for one day and then it was gone, just like it never happened, as the world moved on to examining someone else's life.

One of life's great ironies is that our deepest moments of mental despair can often come as we experience huge success in other areas; it is no coincidence that my first dark moment happened as I was winning medals. With running, there is so much physical and mental pressure on the body and mind. Often the wear and tear can lead to injuries that linger because you can't give them enough time to heal and that in turn creates pressure and worry about not being at the top of your game. I had numerous problems for seven years of my twelve-year career: a stress fracture, a ruptured calf muscle, a torn Achilles tendon, numerous calf tears, glandular fever, tonsillitis, the list goes on. I was emotionally

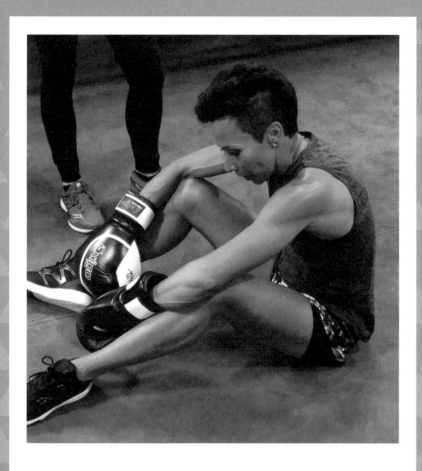

When I first spoke about depression back in 2005, I don't think people wanted to hear it

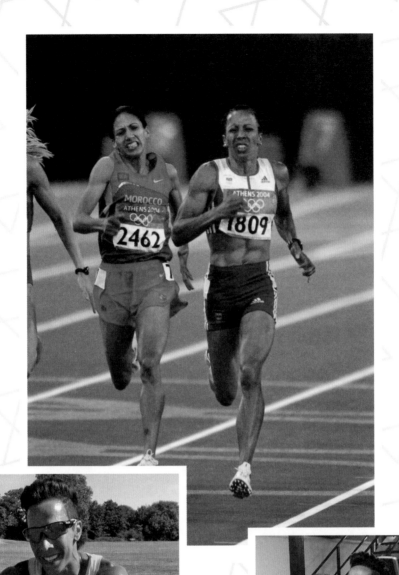

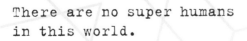

There are no super humans
in this world.

drained and worried about not achieving my ultimate dream.

Like a bolt of lightning in 2003, I was stuck down by an all-consuming, incomprehensible pressure in my head that led me to pick up some scissors and cut myself, not once, twice, or three times, but many times. There I was winning gold in the 800m and 1500m at the Athens Olympic Games in 2004, but in the year before these victories, I had been picking up scissors from my bathroom sink and cutting myself regularly to relieve the anguish I was feeling after being injured. Self-harming was almost a relief. I did it every day. I couldn't see clearly and when I cut myself the first time, it didn't actually seem painful. I used to hide it with make-up and make the cuts in places you couldn't see. It was as if I needed to punish myself for the injuries I had sustained over time. I hated myself and I did not want to be here.

Depression in my eyes is a dark hole with no tunnel and no light. The terrible thing is that, once you have experienced being in that place, it is frighteningly easy to slip back there whenever anything goes wrong. I have been back there many times – I have felt scared of life, when I have been worried about losing my identity and, most devastatingly, when trying to process the death of my mother. *It's an awful place to be.*

I sometimes worry about writing things like this. I am not in any way glorifying my problems, or saying it's okay to do things to yourself, but I also think that being in the public eye means I have an opportunity to make people realise there are no super humans. We all struggle and just want to do our best. Particularly in the sporting world, depression can be seen as a weakness – it seems you are giving your opposition one over on you as you compete against the world's best. We are now in a better place around talking about mental health but we have a long way to go.

The need to perform meant I was screaming inside. It's a pressure-cooker situation and in 2003 it got really bad. I was pushing my body to the extreme in an environment where every tenth of a second counted. Professional running is like being permanently strapped in to a rollercoaster –the highs of wins and medals and the lows of injuries and self-loathing – it felt there was nothing steady in my life and no one to really see what was going on inside. In sport you can go to physiotherapy to treat your obvious injuries, but you are rarely asked how you feel, so you keep it in.

Depression left me floundering and trying desperately to grab on to any hope that could keep me on track. Up until the point I became ill, my life had been one of structure and I had always known where I was, what was coming next and what I wanted.

I grew up in Kent and joined the army a month before I was 18. In the forces and then in sport, there was always a rigid structure to what was expected of me. Facing injury sparked a deep fear inside – I was terrified I would lose that certainty and sense of identity – and it made me feel really vulnerable. I was at the peak of my career but in emotional turmoil – stress and pressure can cause extreme reactions and our bodies and minds need nurturing, not punishing. It is about emotional wellbeing and I wasn't paying any attention to mine.

I can now identify my feelings and thoughts, by the following:

>> **MY MOTIVATION:**
I am generally super motivated, determined and driven to succeed, if I am feeling low then I start to get disheartened and fed up with everything I am doing, which makes me feel overwhelmed. The first thing I do is step away from what I am doing and ask myself what I actually *want* to be doing. It can be as simple as setting a new goal with a narrower focus – or swapping taks for something that feels more achievable at that particular moment.

>> **MY ENERGY LEVELS:**
I get called a Duracell bunny by friends and, to be honest, most of the time this is me. I am on autopilot, can't sit down for long, and am always wanting to travel and get involved with things. This probably only calms down when I have completely overcooked it and gone too far, usually combined with a lack of sleep, not eating well and doing too much.

>> **MY ATTITUDE TO WORK AND PEOPLE:**
I am a very positive person in front of everyone I meet in my working life. I love motivating and encouraging people to be the best version of themselves. I also think I am a 'speak to people how you wish to be spoken to' kind of person and I'm not great when people give me a bad attitude or are rude to others. I believe I am a pretty nice person, but if I am riled I give as much as I get. I would say this trait is one I have learned to control.

I hate being let down or taken for granted; treat me with respect and you will get it back in bundles, take away my trust and I am not good at dealing with the disrespect that comes with it. That said, there are a lot of circumstances where I just think: 'Walk away' or breathe and let it go over my head.

The depression, the self-harm, I didn't talk about any of it as I didn't want to seem weak. I had endless conversations with myself: 'How do I get out of this?' and 'What has happened to me? Where have I gone?'

›› MY ERRATIC EATING PATTERNS:

I am all about balance. I am not good at healthy-only living, but I do know when enough is enough and the control button needs to be pressed.

When I am feeling low I don't have much energy and temptation sneaks up on me, so I nibble on unhealthy snacks as a 'quick fix'. Unhelpfully, I am an all-or-nothing kind of person. If I am stressed I will sit and eat a whole bag of chocolates, however big it is. Conversely, if I am upset I can go without eating all day. Neither of these really helps me feel better but, at that moment, I don't really care. The other side of this is when I am 'on it', I am really good at eating the right balance of food for my daily living and training demands. SO much of that depends on your food intake and exercise pattern.

›› MY SLEEPING PATTERNS:

I am not a good sleeper and this is something I am still trying to work on. I am not sure if it's a combination of anxiety, because I have been in a place of turmoil since my mother passed away, and the fact that I have upped my exercise to mad levels and my adrenaline is sky-high in the evenings. But I am trying different methods of relaxation, like using a spray infused with lavender, vetivert and camomile – this combination is thought to really help calm you, so I have started spaying it on my pillow at night. Sleep teas are recommended so I drink one in bed and I have a salt lamp by the side of my bed. Himalayan salt lamps have natural living proponents and other fans of Himalayan pinksalt lamps (HPS lamps) claim that the negative salt ions released by heating can boost blood flow, improve sleep, increase levels of serotonin in the brain, and calm allergy or asthma symptoms. I am not sure whether my small lamp really gives out such strong vibes, but its worth giving it a go. The other thing that can help is a meditation app.

RUNNING LIFE

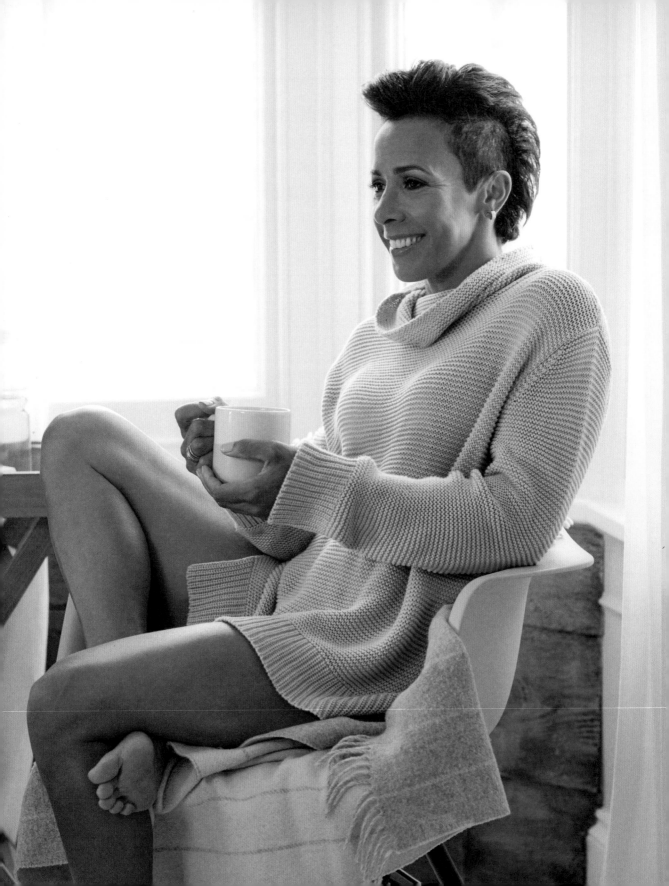

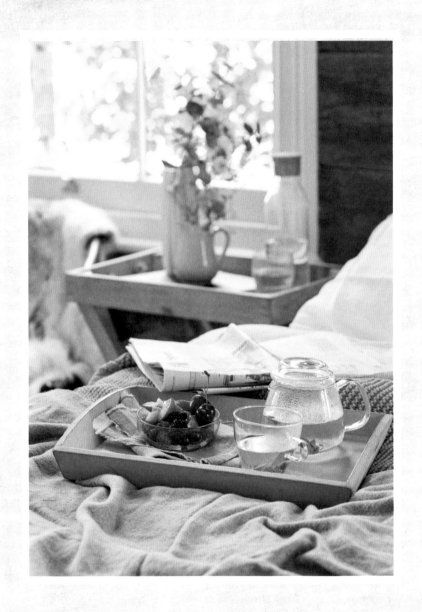

I grew up in the seventies and my mother had me at the young age of 17. At that time she was unable to provide a stable home because her dad (my granddad) did not approve of the fact that, firstly, I was mixed raced and, secondly, she was a single mother. My birth father left way before I turned one and had very little to do with me afterwards and so Mum ended up having to put me in a children's home in Tunbridge Wells.

As we become adults, it is always hard finding out things about our childhoods that we did not know. Even as I write this book, I am experiencing small shocks as I discover more about my time living in the home: who looked after me and, particularly, how long I was there for. I lived there, away from my mum, until I started school but I thought I had left by the time I was three. It is probably easier to have this knowledge now that I am older but I am having to put the pieces together myself as my mother is no longer here for me to ask.

So what can I say about school? Well I loved it for two reasons: sport and my friends! I was not academic at all, always outside the classroom during French because of talking, looking out the window and daydreaming in Maths and English or playing with (Ouija) boards in R.E!

But P.E was something else completely, it was brilliant and I loved everything about it: freedom, fun, expelling excess energy, being part of a team, being good at running and being outside of the classroom gave me a sense of purpose and a name. I believe it only takes one person to make a difference to your life forever. I had some great mates at school who are still my friends to this day. They knew I was obsessed with running throughout. I still remember the moment I went back to school after watching Sebastian Coe win gold in the 1500m at the 1984 Olympic Games in Moscow. I told my friends Kerrie, Lara and Kim that I was going to be an Olympic champion and they said: 'We know you are because that's all you are bloody good at.' That cemented our friendship!

Be aware of yourself, your surroundings and your feelings. Identify with what makes you happy. For me, it's a run to clear my head or a catch-up with my long-term friends.

WHAT'S YOUR HAPPY PLACE?

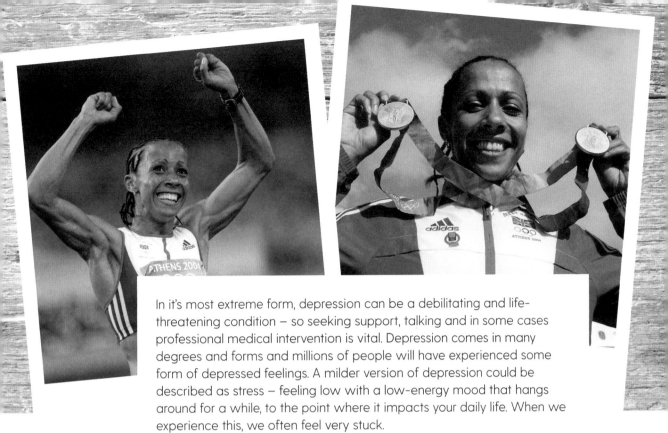

In it's most extreme form, depression can be a debilitating and life-threatening condition – so seeking support, talking and in some cases professional medical intervention is vital. Depression comes in many degrees and forms and millions of people will have experienced some form of depressed feelings. A milder version of depression could be described as stress – feeling low with a low-energy mood that hangs around for a while, to the point where it impacts your daily life. When we experience this, we often feel very stuck.

As humans, we all experience low moods and feel sad at times in our lives. Often we can make sense of why we feel this way (there is an obvious reason for feeling low) and the feelings do pass in time. It is very important for us to notice if this starts to feel different, if the low mood doesn't seem to be shifting and it begins to interfere with life or returns several times.

I first realised I was depressed in conjunction with my self-harming and I knew things were just not right. I was afraid to tell my coach or training partners because I didn't want them to think I was weak or to distract them with my problems in any way. I didn't want to tell my friends or family because I didn't want to worry them.

In the end, the person I confided in hardly spoke English and was a doctor in the mountains of France where I was having a massage. The reason I spoke to her was not because I wanted to, but because I lost the plot, right there on the massage table, and the masseur was worried about this sobbing women lying on her bed. The doctor came in and I just blurted it all out. Talking helped me come to terms with what I was doing and put things into perspective. That chat probably saved my life.

Reasons for depression

Depression varies widely from person to person. Sometimes it occurs in response to a major life event and at other times there seems to be no obvious reason at all. It can be very helpful to explore our feelings of depression to help us try to make sense of why we feel this way, especially if we are feeling stuck, or in the cases where it's hard to put our finger on why we are feeling this way. Some reasons for depression are as follows:

>> **LIFE-CHANGING EVENTS**
Your feelings of depression may have an obvious cause perhaps triggered by a life-changing event. This could be a bereavement, a loss of another kind (see pages 72–78), being the victim of a crime, being bullied, difficulties at work, difficulties in relationships or trying to manage too many responsibilities and demands. For me, my triggers have been: family conflict, leaving the army, finishing my athletics career, difficult relationships and the loss of my mother.

>> **CHILDHOOD**
Through exploring possible reasons for depression, your thoughts may be brought back to your childhood. If you identify with experiences such as a significant loss, abuse of any kind or unsettling experiences then these may have created a vulnerability to depression later in your life. This can very much depend on how you learned to deal with your emotions and cope with difficulties as a child and how much support you received.

It is only as I have got older that I have realised the impact my unstable early life has had on me. I think my reluctance to get to close to people, through fear they will leave me, is definitely a product of my mother having to leave me in the care home as a child. However, I can't necessarily add this as a contributing factor to my depression later in life.

>> **MENTAL HEALTH ILLNESSES & HEALTH PROBLEMS**
It is common for those who are coping with mental health problems to also struggle with depression. Coping with health issues or physical problems can get you down and often lead to feeling depressed, particularly problems that have had a significant effect on your lifestyle, or lead to the loss of activities that you previously enjoyed.

SIGNS OF DEPRESSION

EVERYONE'S EXPERIENCE OF DEPRESSION VARIES, BUT HERE ARE A FEW FEELINGS THAT ARE COMMONLY ASSOCIATED WITH DEPRESSION:

- Low mood, tearful or upset
- Angry or irritable
- Noticing excessive negative thoughts and self-talk
- Low or no confidence
- Guilt
- Lonely or cut off from others
- Loss of joy or happiness in things you previously enjoyed
- In despair or suicidal

HERE ARE SOME OF THE WAYS WE CAN BEHAVE WHEN WE ARE FEELING DEPRESSED:

- Low energy and tiredness
- Unhealthy eating patterns (either eating too little or too much)
- Unable to sleep or sleeping too much
- Avoiding friends, family, social events and activities you previously enjoyed
- Loss of libido
- Forgetfulness and lack of concentration
- Body feels heavy
- Self-harm
- Suicidal thoughts

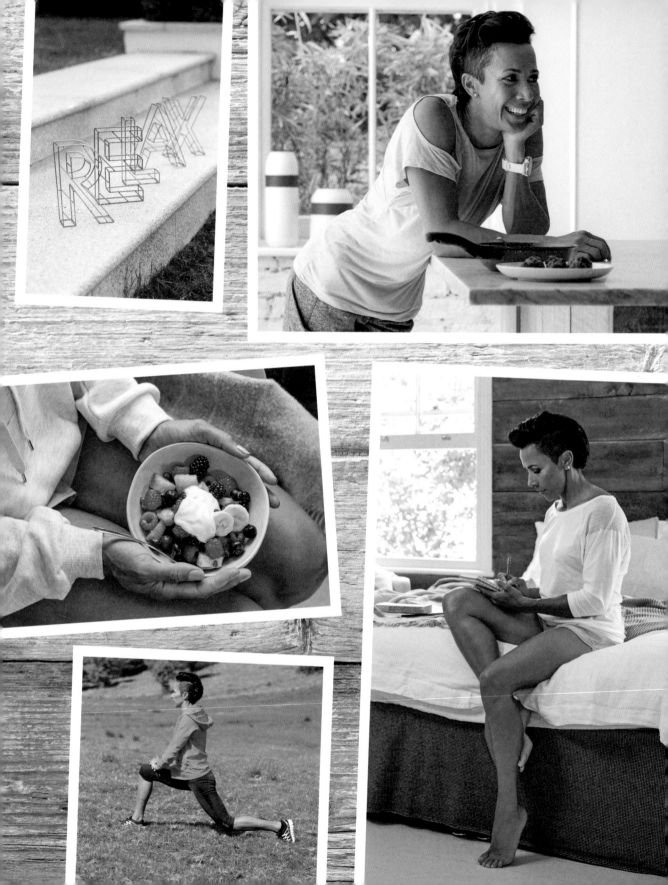

HERE ARE A FEW WAYS IN WHICH YOU CAN BEGIN TO HELP YOURSELF:

>> **SLEEP**

Being unable to sleep or sleeping too much is a common problem when you are depressed. Getting a healthy amount of sleep can significantly improve your mood and give you more energy. Try listening to guided meditation to help you sleep better, or explore alternative therapies. Everyone is different, so if one attempt does not work, try something new.

>> **SELF-CARE ROUTINES**

Taking care of yourself, even in small ways, can help improve your mood. Try to establish routines like soaking in a bath, listening to music, pampering yourself and getting dressed in to something you like wearing even though you might not be going out.

>> **EXERCISE**

Low mood and low energy can be a real challenge to keeping active. However, being active can also significantly improve your mood and boost your feeling of wellbeing. Try starting with gentle exercise like going for a walk, a swim or an exercise class such as yoga or Pilates.

>> **NUTRITION**

Eating well, that is to say a balanced diet and less junk food, will improve your wellbeing, energy levels and feelings. Good food is some of the most important medicine you can give yourself (see pages 150–221).

>> **LISTS – PRACTICAL EXERCISE**

Write a list of things that make you happy or that you see as little treats and start a new routine of doing one of these things every day. Some examples might be: a bubble bath, reading something new from your favourite author, drawing, painting or another creative outlet, a relaxation exercise you enjoy or volunteering. Make a list of things that you would like to try and see if you can do one new thing from your list each week.

>> **STAYING CONNECTED WITH OTHERS**

You can stay connected with others in many ways. If you don't feel up to seeing friends or family, reach out with a text, phone call or email to keep in touch. When you feel up to it, talk to a trusted friend about how you are feeling. It can be a difficult step to take but there is good evidence that talking about how we feel can help to improve how we feel.

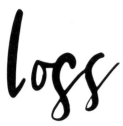

Loss

BEREAVEMENT

Loss through bereavement can feel devastating and can involve extreme emotional pain. Most of us are aware that the death of someone we care about will be followed by a grief process or period of mourning. During this time we may experience a sense of major change in our lives and it can sometimes feel like we are stuck, or at best, making a very slow recovery.

The effects of bereavement can vary from person to person. You might experience a wide range of physical and emotional symptoms as you go through the grief process. These can include extreme sadness, loneliness, sleep problems, depression, stress, anxiety and anger. I have been through all of these during the process of losing my mother.

OTHER LOSSES

We can be seriously impacted by other losses, but unlike bereavement, we can be unaware that we still need to go through a grief process in order to recover. Essentially, any situation that involves an ending is a loss in our life. Even a situation where we have chosen to bring about this ending. We might feel confused as to why we feel so overwhelmed but as soon as we name the experience as a loss we can begin to make sense of the process that is necessary to bring about change and restore balance.

TYPES OF LOSS

- Bereavement
- Ending of a relationship including friendships
- Divorce
- Miscarriage and all pregnancy losses
- Infertility
- Moving house
- Children leaving home
- Redundancy
- Loss of self esteem and confidence
- Loss of your identity
- Leaving a long career
- PTSD (post-traumatic stress disorder)

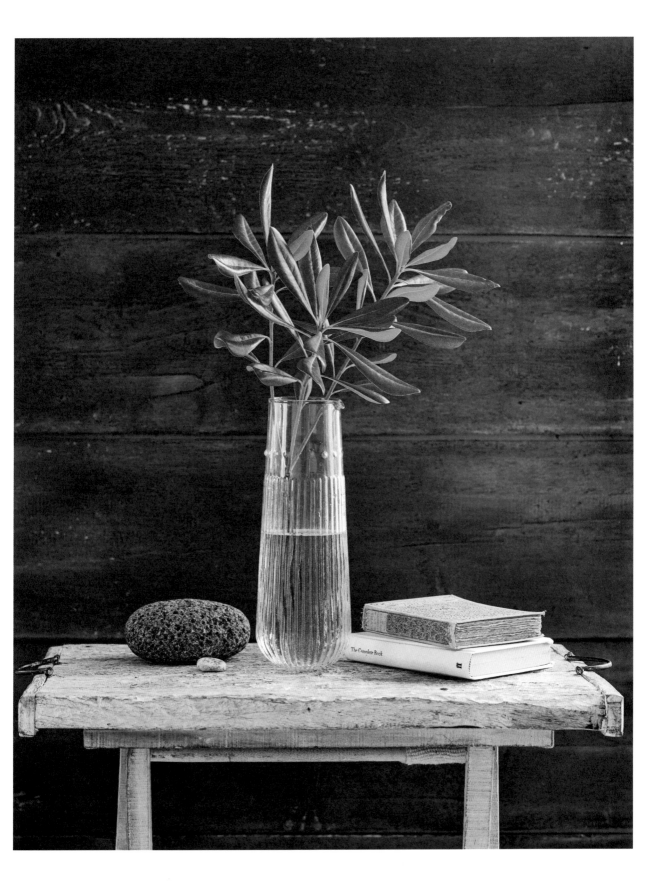

Immediately after experiencing bereavement or loss, you may feel a number of things as a reaction to what you are facing. These reactions can include the following (in no particular order):

>> **SHOCK**
Shock is a powerful reaction to loss. It may take time for you to fully acknowledge what has happened. The effects of loss can be a feeling of numbness, difficulty accepting the situation and feeling disorientated.

When I first found out about my mother's illness it was a huge shock and the last thing any of us expected as my nan, my mum's mum, lived until 98 years old so we always thought mum would be here for that long too. As a sports person, when someone says they have a backache or muscle ache, you immediately think that it's tightness or a posture issue. We found out by chance really when a doctor at the hospital she worked at said he thought she should have a test for myeloma. First of all, I had never heard of it, secondly, it seemed impossible she would have it – how could that be?

>> **PAIN AND DEPRESSION**
Experiencing a loss can be deeply painful and at times overwhelming and distressing. Feelings of depression can affect many people who have experienced loss. You can become very low for a period of time before things feel like they are improving.

>> **ANGER**
Feelings of anger are not unusual. You may feel that the situation you are in is extremely unfair. This can apply to a bereavement if you feel that the person you care about has died before they should have, or you're angry with the person themselves for things that they did/didn't do or say before their death. Other types of loss can very often involve feelings of anger too. You might feel a sense of injustice or feel furious at the way that you have been treated.

>> **LONGING**
Another stage that can happen is a sense of longing for events to have been different. In cases of bereavement or the ending of a relationship you can find yourself longing for the person that is no longer in your life. You may become very preoccupied with thoughts of seeing or hearing them again, including mistaking someone you see when you are out and about, for the person you are longing for.

THE FIVE STAGES OF GRIEF AND LOSS ARE:

1. **Denial and isolation**
2. **Anger**
3. **Bargaining**
4. **Depression**
5. **Acceptance**

PEOPLE WHO ARE GRIEVING DO NOT NECESSARILY GO THROUGH THE STAGES IN THE SAME ORDER, OR EVEN EXPERIENCE ALL OF THEM.

These stages of grief and mourning are universal and are experienced by people from all walks of life, across many cultures. Mourning occurs in response to an individual's own terminal illness, the loss of a close relationship, or the death of a valued human or animal. The five stages of grief were first proposed by Elisabeth Kübler-Ross in her 1969 book *On Death and Dying*.

In our bereavement, we spend different lengths of time working through each step and express each stage with different levels of intensity. The five stages of loss do not necessarily occur in any specific order. We often move between stages before achieving a more peaceful acceptance of death. Many of us are not afforded the luxury of time to achieve this final stage of grief.

Throughout each stage, a common thread of hope emerges: *As long as there is life, there is hope. As long as there is hope, there is life.* The death of my mother inspired me to evaluate my own feelings of mortality.

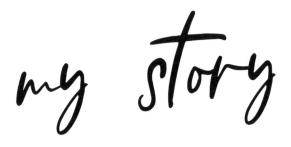

my story

I HAVE SUFFERED A FEW DIFFERENT FORMS OF LOSS AND I WANT TO SHARE ONE OF MY STORIES WITH YOU.

- ## THE ARMY

I served in the British Army for nine and a half years. First as a heavy goods vehicle driver when I joined aged 17 and later as a Physical Training instructor. I craved independence, a career and a way of belonging. I had a great career in the army building strong relationships with other soldiers from around the UK and the world. The bonds that you make are second to none and the friendships can last a lifetime, as some of mine have.

I don't think I really appreciated the lifestyle I led, a roof over my head, a guaranteed monthly wage, friendships that will never be broken because of circumstances that were shared. I loved being in the army, it was part of me that made sense. Driven to succeed, challenged to be better than others, respect, values, integrity and support.

I left the military in 1997 because I had also become an international athlete winning medals for my country, whilst serving my country. What I probably didn't factor in was the effect leaving would have on me.

It was, at the time, one of the hardest decisions I'd made. At the age of 27 years old I gave up a career I loved, something I was good at and that was secure. But I had to.

I only now appreciate the powerful effect of the army on my life, my upbringing as a teenager, my strength of character and the friendships I have made. Some of my army friends are very much in my life now and I want to take the opportunity to recogise them: Sue (Chalkie) Dawson, Tremay (Dobo) Dobson, Jackie (Jacs) Gilchrist, Jaci (Staff) Langhorn, Mark (still young) Bennett and Emma (you will carry the goal post) Taylor. I value their friendship, their support and their trust so much.

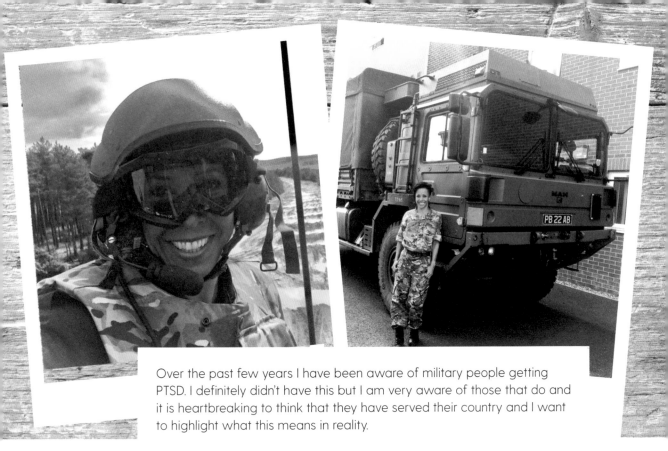

Over the past few years I have been aware of military people getting PTSD. I definitely didn't have this but I am very aware of those that do and it is heartbreaking to think that they have served their country and I want to highlight what this means in reality.

My career was a massive ending for me because I was scared of what would happen. Would I ever get a job again if my athletics didn't go well? What if my athletics career went horribly wrong? I became anxious about everything, some things which I could not change, but, when the fear descended, I tried to think positively about what I did have. I was a talented runner pursuing a dream. Many people never take a leap of faith and, instead, live with regrets.

By the time I was 26, I ensured that I was financially stable by buying a house back in Kent (in case it all went wrong!), near my family but not so close that I felt I would be going backwards as I didn't want to lose my independence. My family were really supportive of my athletics career, having already seen me become Commonwealth champion and a European and World Championship medallist.

At the time I was lucky enough to be fully engaged in my athletics career and was distracted by a bad injury I sustained at the 1997 World Championships in Athens, rupturing my calf and tearing my Achilles tendon, so I had something for my mind to focus on. I was also given an MBE by the Queen for services to the British Army which I am so honoured to receive. I left with my head held up high. But it was a loss to my identity.

• LEAVING ATHLETICS

Sport may create heroes, and now celebrities, but a massive number of athletes lose their identity when they finish competingand that definitely happened to me.

It's easy to tell someone: 'I'm an Olympian,' because that's what you do, that's your career, but when you retire and you start saying 'former this' or 'I used to do that', it changes you aś a person and also has an impact on the people around you. Your friends and family have always known you as a focused, driven, high-achieving person who gets up at this time, eats at that time, trains for this amount of time – it totally defines who you are and how you interact with them. It is front and centre of every choice you make, and when that is gone, it is hard.

Suddenly no longer having a goal was a difficult experience. My dream for 20 years was to be an Olympic champion. That was my driving force, without that I was left wondering: 'What's the next thing for me to aim for?' When you have been great at something, how do you become as good at something new? It opened the floodgates to the question: 'Is "good" good enough?'

I have a need to be excellent and lots of other sports people share that trait. The problem is how to measure it once you stop competing. With sport it's easy: you get the medal or you don't, you get the time or you don't. It's not as easy to measure your day-to-day successes when they don't involve competing. Some athletes have planned for retirement and prepared their next career in advance, others get injured and it's a premature decision.

There have always been a lot of questions about where to go next in my life, though not always immediate answers. A huge amount of sports people say: 'I don't know who I am any more' once they aren't competing. Coming to terms with how life is going to be once you leave behind a sporting structure is always hard, but over the years (and with the benefit of age and experience), I have started to ensure that I ask myself some questions about my new life (see opposite). This is one of the reasons I set up my charity, the Dame Kelly Holmes Trust.

QUESTIONS I ASK ABOUT MY NEW LIFE . . .

1 AM I ENJOYING WHAT I AM DOING?
If not then change is a must for happiness. I was not enjoying working out of an office I had in Kent whilst running an education company that I owned, as it was not inspiring me any more so I decided to close up and move on to new things and that gave me a new lease of life.

2 AM I MAKING THE MOST OF OPPORTUNITIES?
Open your eyes to things that are there for you to try and experience as you never know where it will take you. If an opportunity comes to me then I will look at it and, if I take it up, I give it my best shot. Like most things in life I would rather know then live with the 'if only'.

3 WHAT CAN I CHANGE?
Depending on what you want to change take the first steps by writing down what it is that needs fixing and have small targets to change what you can. Sometimes I ask for help, or I just have the foresight, determination and guts to say: 'Right, we need to change'.

mindset

MINDSET IS KEY TO SUCCESS IN ANY ASPECT OF YOUR LIFE, AND YET LOOKING AFTER IT CAN BE THE THING THAT COMES LAST ON OUR TO-DO LIST.

It is a complex and tricky area, so I have tried my best to show the different ways that certain situations can sabotage and unsettle our mental equilibrium. But even if you suffer from any of the conditions in this section, remember that you can still be in control.

This book is about 360-degree health and happiness and that isn't just good nutrition and lifting weights – it is about having the knowledge to know when your mind is fragile and needs an extra helping hand. We are all unique and the going gets tough for us all, some people just need more help than others. I have been there and there's certainly no shame in that. I look at what I have achieved and I am proud. I believe things happen for a reason. If you have an opportunity come to you in life, you have a choice: go for it, or never know. I have always said I will never live with the 'if only' as 'if only' is too late.

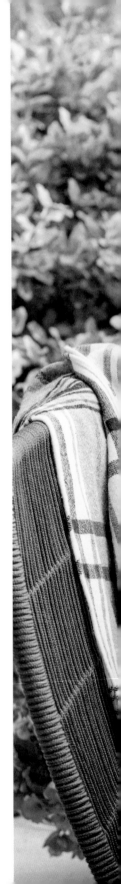

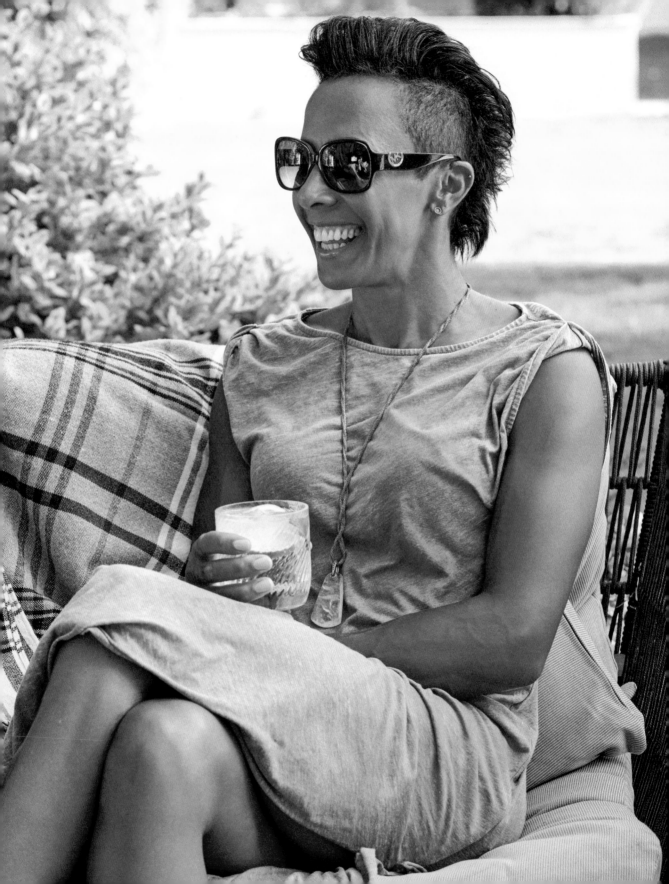

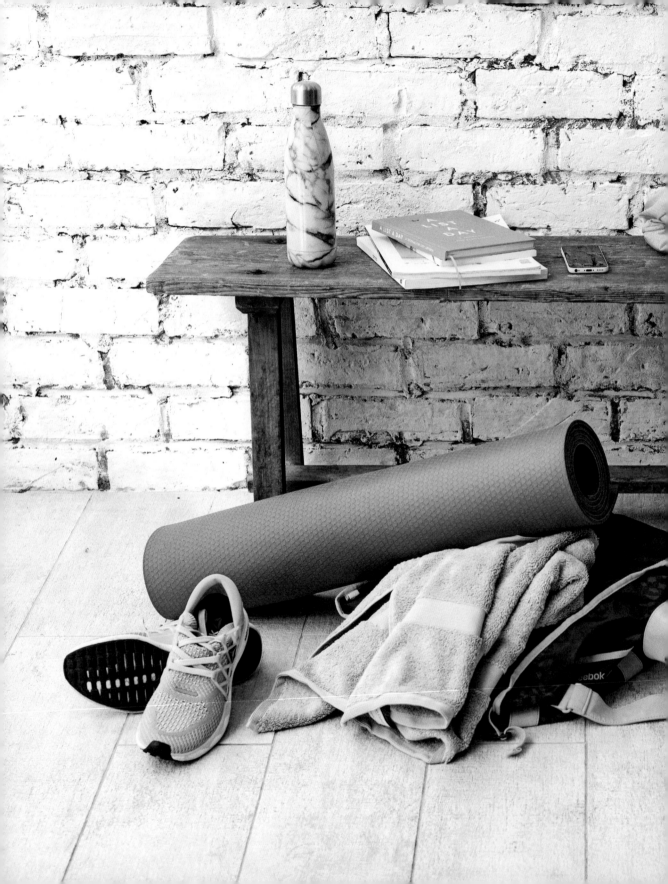

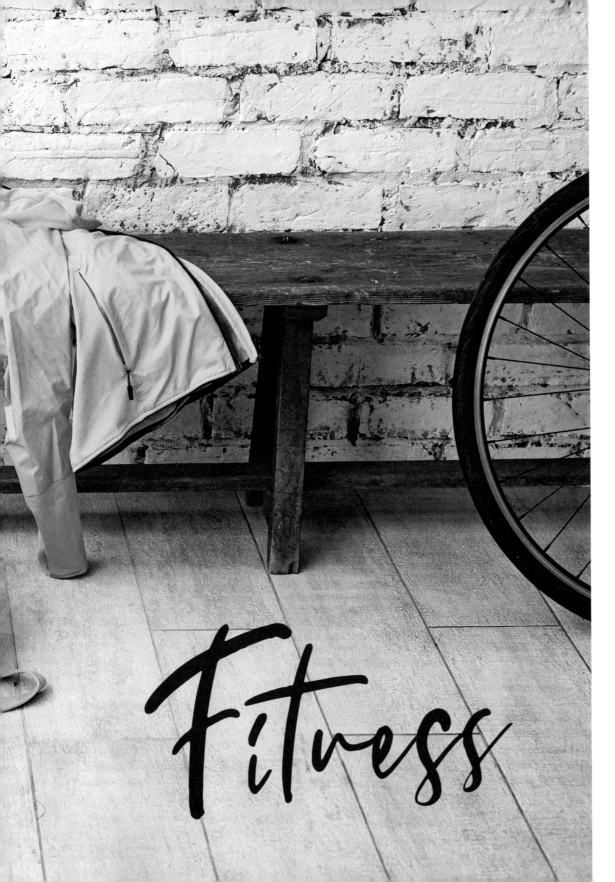

Fitness

Champion's Mind

I'D LIKE TO THINK I HAVE A PRETTY GOOD UNDERSTANDING OF WHAT IT TAKES TO BE A CHAMPION.

I have certainly always believed that people 'win' because they have the right mental attitude. In my mind, it is all about believing anything is possible but that doesn't automatically mean everyone is a winner. Because when two people have the same qualifications, experience in the workplace or time and distance on the track, it's the mental attitude, focus and self-belief that can set them apart.

Now, when we are talking fitness and sport, this is so true. Anyone can go to the gym and train if they choose to. But it's all about making the choice to be healthy in the first place – deciding to do the best by our body starts us on the path to fitness and consistency. We all know it's easy to say 'no', or 'I can't', but no one will do it for you – you have to want to be your own champion.

Desire, wish and aspiration help you focus on what you really want. Having a long-term goal, whatever that is to you, is key to forming new habits and being the best you can be. This section will focus on running but also on everyday fitness – we will look at all aspects of training, including motivation to start your training programme, tips on how to maintain your new way of life, goal setting and tracking your progress. I want you to have solid foundations and the desire to improve every day.

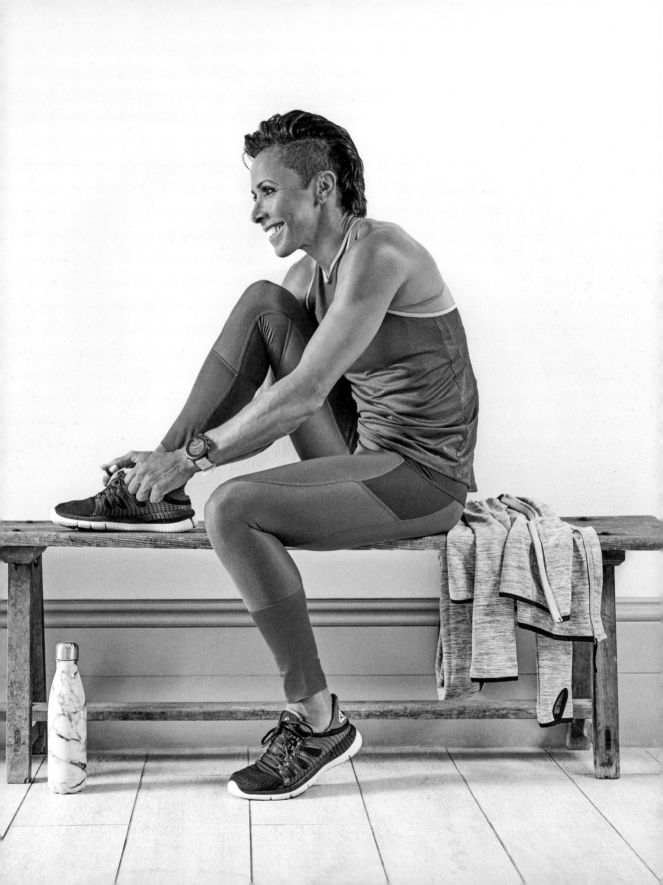

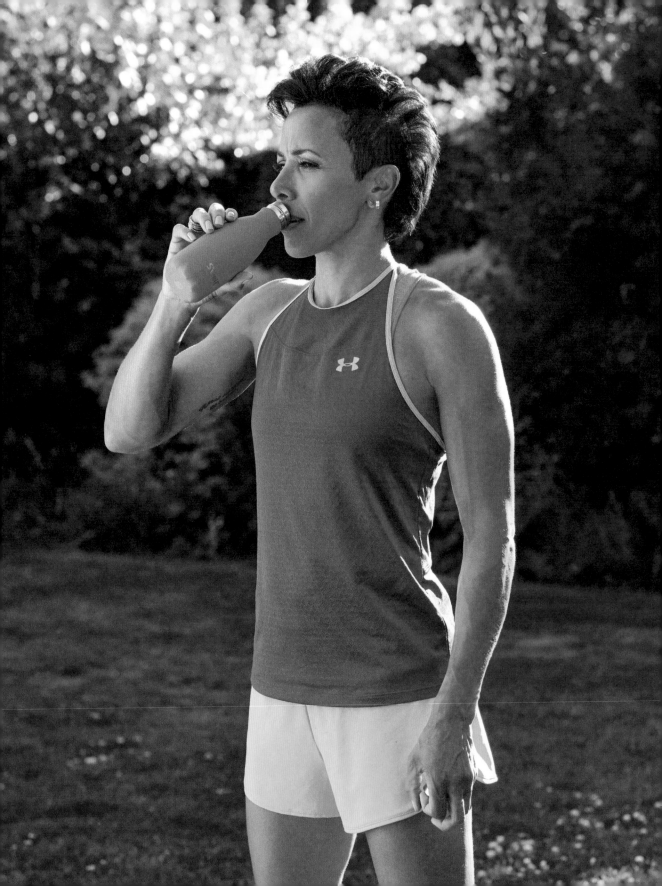

TRAINING TIPS

Whether it is general exercise or running, it is all about creating a routine that works for you and, once you have that in place, you will be well on your way. But getting started is the hardest bit – how do you build new habits if you don't know where or how to begin? Here are some tips to help you create the perfect training routine:

---

1. MOTIVATION:
Before you start anything new you have to want to actually start! Depending on how busy I am there is always a moment where training can fall down the priority list – we are all guilty of that, but the key is making time in your diary that cannot be missed.

2. HAVE A GOAL:
What do you want to achieve with your training? There is nothing worse than walking into the gym and not having a clue what to do, or setting off for a run with no idea what your performance goal is. Start every workout with a plan, know how long you are training for and what you need to achieve out of that session – is it a heavier weight, a few more reps or another mile on your running distance?

3. TRACK YOUR PROGRESS:
It is important to keep notes or a diary of what you achieve each week so you can see your fitness progress, even if, initially, the changes seem small.

4. BE REALISTIC:
Changes to your body or your fitness levels won't happen overnight. You have to commit to eating honestly and training regularly.

5. HYDRATE:
Your body has a much easier job of giving you its best when you are hydrated. Your muscles repair quicker, your metabolism is faster, your circulation and digestion are better. Drink at least 2 litres of water a day; 3 litres if you are training.

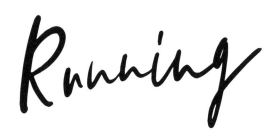

Running

YOU MIGHT BE THINKING: 'OF COURSE KELLY KNOWS HOW TO RUN, SHE HAS WON MEDALS! BUT HOW IS SOMEONE LIKE ME EVER GOING TO BE ABLE TO DO IT THE WAY SHE DOES?'

The truth is that you are not, but you can run to the best of your ability. As much as running is the most accessible form of exercise you can do, it's like anything: if you want to progress you have to look at all aspects of your performance.

You get out what you put in and to run well, you have to be fit; to be fit, you have to train. To run better it is about becoming stronger and having good stability – that in turn will help you stay injury free and you will see progress quicker. This section will show you how to train various parts of your body in order to perform at the top of your game. No matter what kind of runner you are, doing a variety of training will bring huge benefits.

I started running when I was 12 years old after my PE teacher, Miss Debbie Page, convinced me to be part of the school cross-country team (something that did not appeal to me at all, as my vision of cross country was always cold, wet, muddy, windy and hard work – which it was!).

But Debbie got her way and I was in the team. I remember the day clearly, as I turned up in a white airtex (see-through) PE shirt, skirt, high-knee white socks and white plimsole shoes. I came second in my first race against the best girl in Kent for our age and it was that moment that changed me. I hated coming second and my competitive nature was born, I was determined to win my next race and all my races from then on. For me there was no point doing it if I wasn't the best out there.

Later that year, Debbie called my mother to take me to Tonbridge Athletics Club in Kent. I went on to win my first English School Championship in Plymouth for the 1500m aged 13. That was it, I was hooked on running.

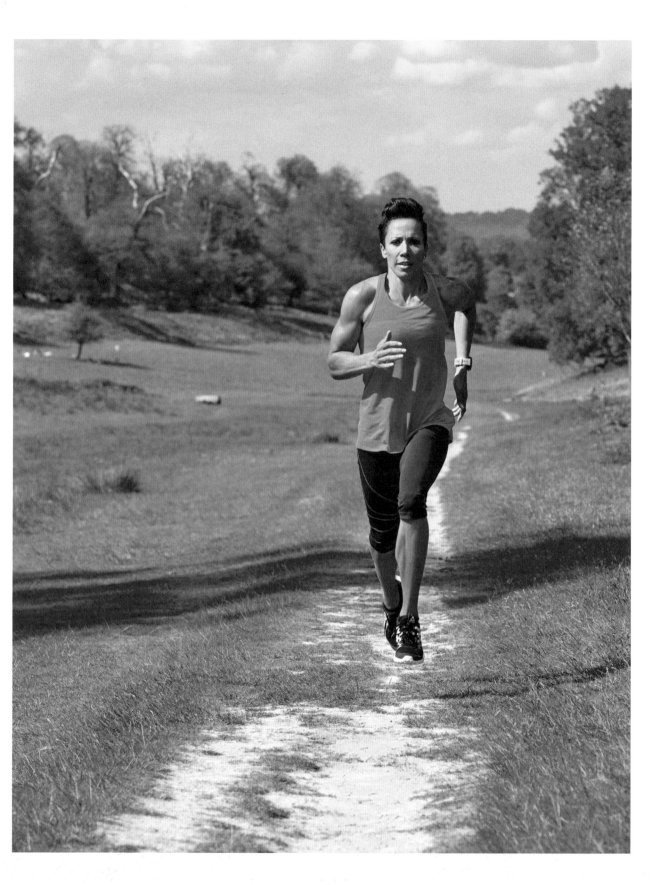

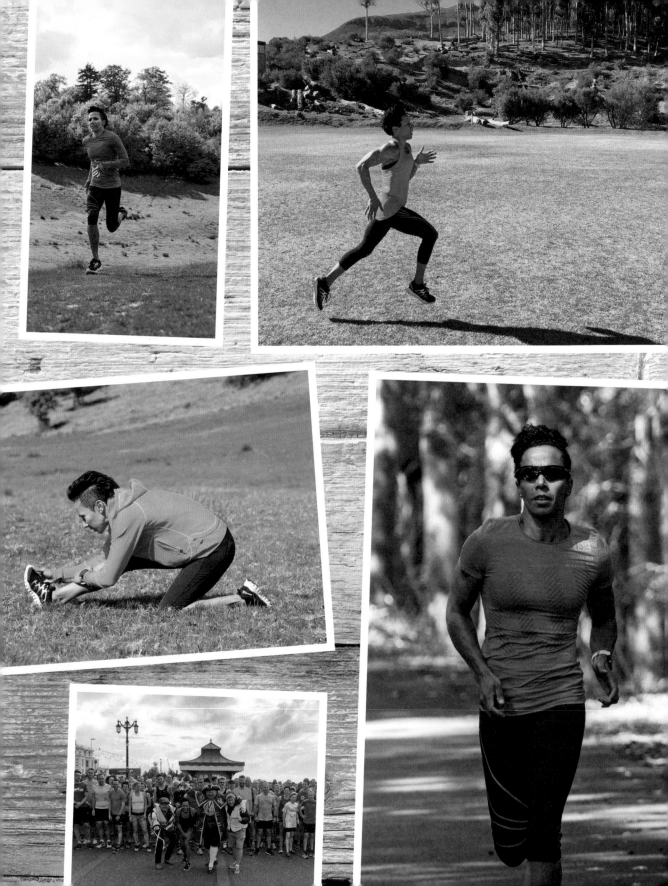

I am a massive fan of the parkrun movement because it's for anyone and everyone. No matter what your age, size, shape, ability, background, we all turn up for the same reason: to complete a 5km.

Running has been part of me for the majority of my life and now it helps me with every aspect of my daily life – it's the thing that brings me joy, it's the thing I turn to in the dark times and it provides a lot of the happy times. Running is free and accessible to anyone – you don't need a gym membership to do it and it doesn't matter about your ability, it's about setting your own pace and rhythm. You can put your headphones on, be inspired and forget your troubles.

I am a massive fan of the parkrun movement because it's for anyone and everyone. No matter what your age, size, shape, ability, background, we all turn up for the same reason: to complete a 5km.

I think we all should have something which takes us to our happy place. These days, running gives me freedom, headspace, confidence, fitness and is part of my lifestyle rather than a career. It's an amazing form of exercise and works your whole body as well as being good for the mind.

The 'Run Better' section (pages 132–150) will give you training and recovery tips and also help you identify your running style. It's about making improvements that will help maximise your ability. You will also learn how to strengthen your body using other forms of exercise – the stronger you are, the better your running experience.

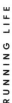

Effective ways to get the most out of your running

>> **CARDIOVASCULAR EXERCISE**
such as HIIT, running, cycling or dancing, exercises your heart and lungs, increasing the efficiency with which your body supplies oxygen to its muscles. As a result, your body's endurance and stamina will gradually increase (and its fatigue levels decrease) with cardiovascular exercise.

>> **LONG-DISTANCE RUNNING OR ENDURANCE RUNNING**
is a form of continuous running over distances of at least 5 miles/8km. Physiologically, it is largely aerobic in nature and requires stamina as well as mental strength. Long distance running can also be used as a means to improve cardiovascular health.

>> **SPEED-ENDURANCE**
is the ability to prolong the amount of time where a near maximal speed can be maintained. If you're running on the road, find a hilly route to run once every week or two. Use an interval programme on the treadmill or create your own speed-endurance workout by increasing the pace for one minute and then recovering for 2–3 minutes, and repeat.

>> **TEMPO RUN**
is a faster-paced workout also known as a lactate-threshold, LT, or threshold run. Tempo pace is often described as 'comfortably hard'. Tempo running improves a crucial physiological variable for running success: our metabolic fitness.

>> **INTERVAL TRAINING**
also known as interval workouts or interval runs, are short, intense efforts followed by equal or slightly longer recovery time. Serious athletes have long known about the benefits of high-intensity interval training – alternating periods of short, intense anaerobic exercise with less intense recovery periods.

Intervals differ from tempo run workouts, mainly because you will have a break between each repetition. Your pace during intervals should also be faster than your tempo run pace. Intervals are a great way to increase your speed endurance and running form.

TWO EXAMPLE INTERVAL SESSIONS

Warm up for 10 minutes, run for 2 minutes at a hard pace, followed by 2-3 minutes of easy jogging or walking to get your heart rate down, repeat 4/6 times or, depending on your distance, up to 10 times.

For middle distance runners, one of my favourite track sessions when I was competing in the 800m and 1500m was 8 x 200m with a 200m jog for recovery and these were done at about 90% max speed. My pace was between 26-28 seconds per 200m. My personal best for 800m was 1:56.21.

>> **FARTLEK**

means 'speed play' and is a form of interval or speed training that can improve your running speed and endurance. Fartlek running involves varying your pace throughout your run, alternating between fast efforts and slow jogs. It improves speed and muscular endurance.

>> **HILL TRAINING**

can be done on an incline treadmill, in a park or even up a hilly street. The fast pace builds speed, but it's the hill that provides the strength benefit. Running up an incline places the same demand on your muscles as weight training – your glutes, quads, hamstrings, and calves must 'lift' you up the slope – but they're more specific to running. Running uphill is an intense activity that activates the entire body.

>> **SPRINTING**

naturally increases the body's short-term endurance strength and muscle tone by improving your muscles' ability to burn glucose through your anaerobic pathways. Through sprinting and speed training exercises, the body increases its ability to store oxygen, which helps the muscles function in all forms of exercise.

Training to be fit for running:

CORE

Whether running for fun, fitness, or to be fast, efficiency is key. A strong core helps runners with their stability, balance, posture and overall control. Core strength training reinforces the way that your pelvis, abs, hips and lower back work together.

- CIRCUIT TRAINING basically means that you perform one exercise right after another with zero rest. Circuit training is good for cardio and strength.

- HIIT (High Intensity Interval Training) is a workout is where you have intervals of rest plus intervals of maximum effort. HIIT is good for endurance and burning fat quickly.

Core exercises are an important part of a well-rounded fitness programme. Aside from occasional sit-ups and push-ups, however, core exercises are often neglected. Still, it pays to get your core muscles — the muscles around your trunk and pelvis — in better shape.

A common misconception is that exercising your core simply means working your abdominal muscles. Core exercises also strengthen your hips, back and all muscles in the midsection of the body. The core is your centre and where all body movements begin. As for all strength workouts, always monitor your form and make sure you're maintaining good posture during each exercise.

HIIT

Body-weight training. This will test both your aerobic and anaerobic fitness. Here's a challenge for you:

- Do as many high knee sprints (page 105) as you can in 20 seconds

- **Rest for 10 seconds**

- Do as many squats (page 107) as you can in 20 seconds

- **Rest for 10 seconds**

- Do as many press-ups (page 116) you can in 20 seconds

- **Rest for 10 seconds**

- Do as many burpees (page 109) as you can in 20 seconds

- **Rest for 10 seconds**

- Do as many Russian twists (page 99) as you can in 20 seconds

- **Rest for 10 seconds**

- Do as many jump squats (page 108) as you can in 20 seconds

- **Rest for 1–2 minutes**

- Repeat the circuit 2–3 times

- Finish the session with a 10-minute cool down

- Record your result in your diary/journal then, during your next session, aim to beat your record

CORE EXERCISES

A Perform 3 sets of 8-12 reps. Hold for 20–60 seconds.

B Rest for 60 seconds between rounds.

C Incorporate these exercises into your routine 2-3 x per week (rest for up to 48 hours in between sessions).

D Make sure you do warm-up exercises first for approximately 10-15 minutes.

E This workout is great after a run or on your gym days.

Here is my 30-day plank challenge

- Start with a basic plank, then for the variations, choose two options from MY FAVOURITE EIGHT PLANK EXERCISES (pages 100–103) and mix it up. (*If you can't sustain the total time then have short break until you have done the total time required.*) This can be done as an extra to your normal training and could be performed after your session.

- **DAY 1** start with a 20-second basic plank and 2 x 10-second variations.

- Add 10 seconds to the basic (*and variation*) planks each day, rest for one day every five days.

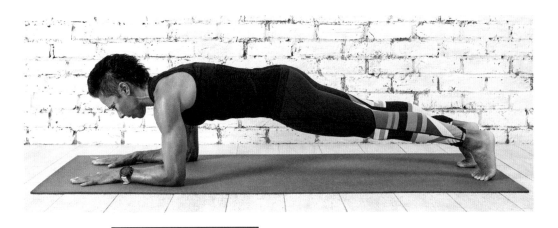

BASIC PLANK

1. The basic plank is one of the best exercises for core conditioning but it also works your glutes and hamstrings, supports proper posture, and improves balance.

2. Place your forearms on the floor with the elbows aligned below the shoulders, your arms parallel to the body and about shoulder-width apart.

3. From the side your arms should form a 90-degree angle. Step your feet back, one at a time. Maintain a straight line from your heels through to the top of your head, looking down at the floor and slightly in front of your hands. Draw in your abs and tighten your glutes – hold.

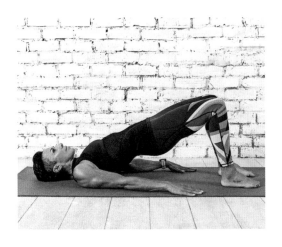

BRIDGE

1. Lie on your back and start to activate your abs. Keep your lower back flat against the floor. Bend your knees at a 90-degree angle with your feet flat on the floor. Your arms can just rest right by your side, palms facing down.

2. Lift your hips and engage your glutes. Push your feet into the floor as you lift your hips. Hold.

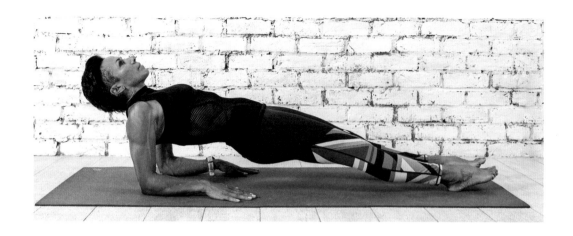

BACK PLANK

1. Start by sitting on the floor with your legs out in front of you.

2. Rest up on your elbows, with your fingers pointing towards your hips. Then push up and lift your body until it forms a straight line from head to toe.

3. Keep your arms in a 90-degree angle and legs straight. Brace your abs.

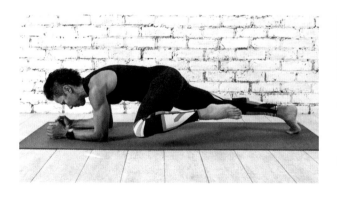

HIGH PLANK KNEE-TO-ELBOW

1. Start out in a basic plank position (see page 97).

2. Engage your glutes and activate the core to keep your back straight. Your shoulders and hips should be in a straight line.

3. Bring your left knee to the outside of your left elbow. Repeat on the opposite side.

RUSSIAN TWIST

1. Sit on the floor with your knees bent. Lean back slightly, keeping your back straight.

2. Pick up a weight or a medicine ball and hold it at chest level, then twist to the right, with the weight or ball.

3. Hold then rotate to the other side. For a more advanced workout use a heavier weight or medicine ball and lift your feet off the floor.

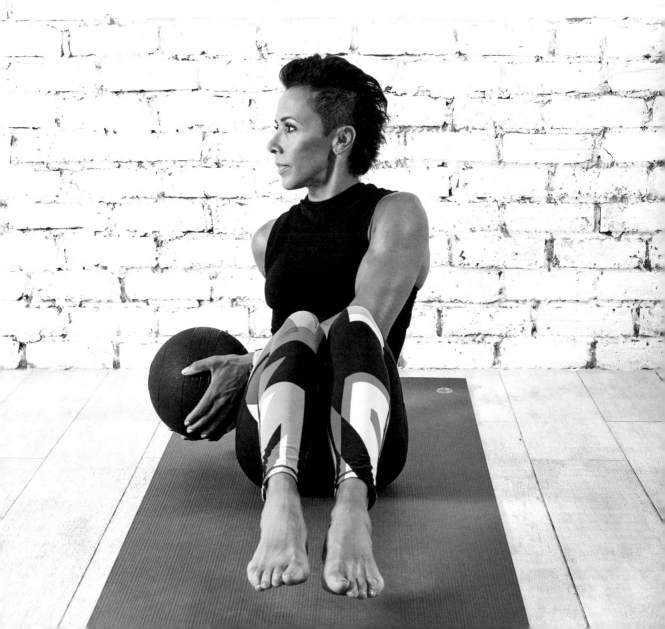

MY FAVOURITE EIGHT PLANK EXERCISES

The plank is one of the best exercises for core conditioning. It also works your glutes and hamstrings, supports proper posture and improves balance.

 BASIC PLANK (ADVANCE TO BALL PLANK)
Place your forearms on the ground with the elbows aligned below the shoulders, your arms parallel to the body and about shoulder-width apart.

From the side your arms should form a 90-degree angle (see page 97).

Step your feet back, one at a time, whilst maintaining a straight line from your heels through the top of your head. Make sure you are looking down at the floor and slightly in front of your hands. Then tighten your abs and glutes. Hold for as long as you can. Don't forget to breathe!

 SIDE PLANK (ADVANCE TO LEG LIFT)
Lying on your right side, lift your body so your weight is propped up on your forearm and the side of your right foot (or, stagger both feet to modify).

There should be a straight diagonal line from your head to your feet. (a) Hold steady, engaging the core muscles. Or, for an even greater challenge, complete 10 lateral leg raises, by slowly lifting your top leg to a 45-degree angle and lowering it back down to the start position. (b) Switch to the left side and repeat.

 BACK PLANK
Start by sitting on the floor with your legs out in front of you. Rest up on your elbows, with your fingers pointing towards your hips. Then push up and lift your body until it forms a straight line from head to toe. Keep your arms in a 90-degree angle and legs straight. Brace your abs (see page 98).

 BALANCE PLANKS
Start by lying on your stomach and prop your weight up on your forearms and toes. (a) Keep a straight line from your head to your feet and hold this position, making sure your abs, glutes, and lower back are engaged. (b) Simultaneously lift the right leg and the left arm, hold for 2–3 seconds, and switch. You could make this easier by lifting one leg or one arm at a time.

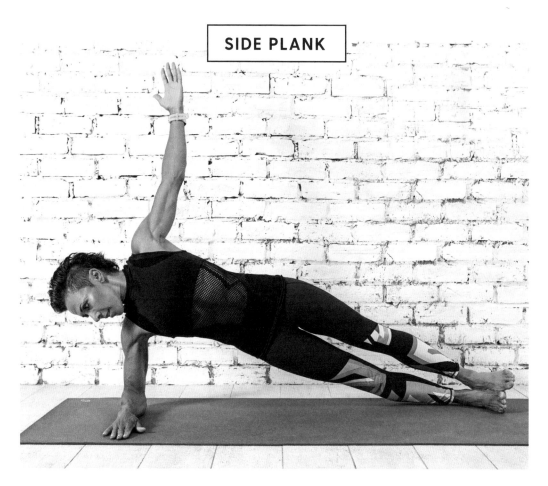

SIDE PLANK

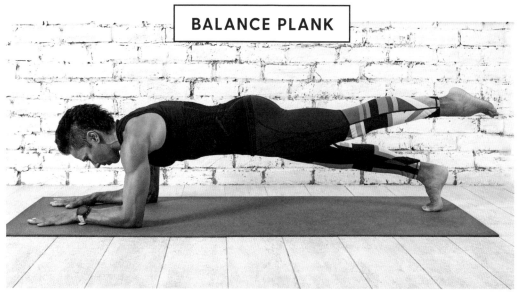

BALANCE PLANK

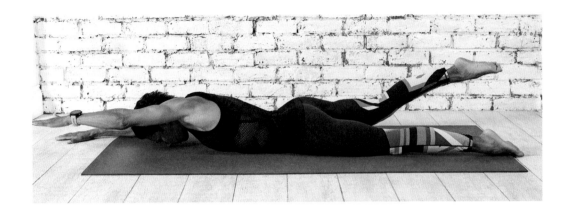

5 SUPERMAN

Lie on your front, then raise your arms, legs and chest off of the floor and hold for 2 seconds. Or lift the opposite arm and leg for a variation.

TIP: Draw your abs in and squeeze your glutes to get the best results from this exercise.

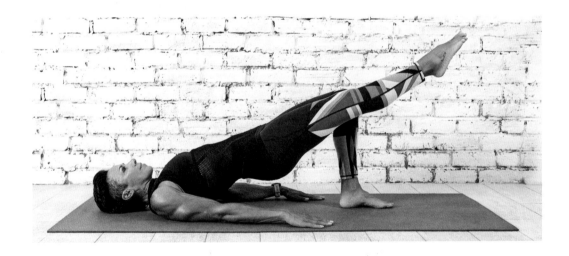

6 SINGLE-LEG GLUTE BRIDGE

Lie on your back with your legs bent and feet flat on the floor. Lift your hips so there is a straight line from your shoulders to your knees. (a) Extend one leg straight out, hold for a few seconds, then place it back down on the floor and repeat on the other side. (b) Make sure your hips don't dip and your bum doesn't sag to the floor during the movement.

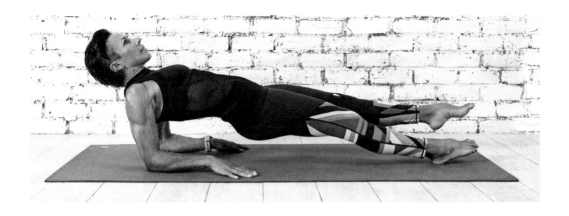

7 ONE-LEG BACK PLANK

Lie on your back with your weight on your elbows and heels .Lift your hips, and keep a straight line from your toes to your shoulders (see Back Plank, page 98). (a) Next, maintaining a solid core and not breaking at the waist, lift your left leg 20cm off the floor and hold for 2–3 seconds. (b) Repeat with the opposite leg.

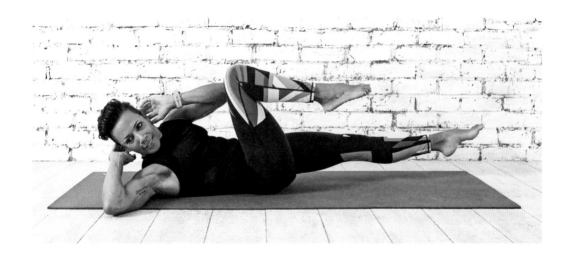

8 MODIFIED BICYCLE

Lie on your back and raise your right leg to a 90-degree angle. Your thigh should be perpendicular to your torso and your shin parallel to the ground. (a) Next, lift your left leg about 7.5cm off the floor, hold for a few seconds, then switch legs. (b) Make sure your lower back is in a neutral position during the entire exercise. You can put your hands in the small of your back to get a flat back.

LEGS

Strong legs are key to running performance. Bodyweight training stabilises the joints, strengthens connective tissues, and improves balance. Adding bodyweight training to your fitness regime will help you improve your running endurance and prevent pain and injury. These first two exercises are drill exercises that improve your co-ordination and conditioning.

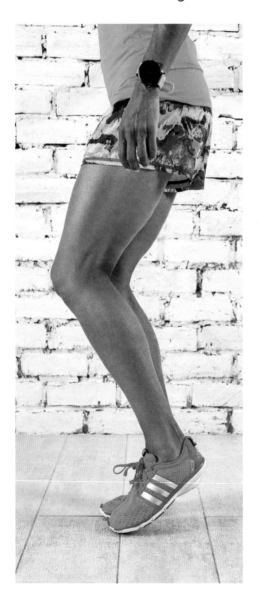

FAST FEET

Improves your running cadence (how many steps you take a minute) by teaching your leg muscles (hamstrings mostly) to fire faster and your feet to turn over quicker.

1. Stand with your knees slightly bent.

2. Run on the spot on your toes, bringing the toes no more that 2–3cm off the ground.

3. Keep the emphasis on speed of movement.

4. Aim for 3 sets of 20–30 seconds.

HIGH KNEES

1. Stand tall.

2. Lift your knees to waist height while landing lightly – but quickly – on the balls of your feet, taking fast, powerful strides.

3. Pump your arms as if you were sprinting.

4. Aim for 3 sets of 10–15 seconds. This drill will elevate your heart rate and fatigue your lower legs quickly.

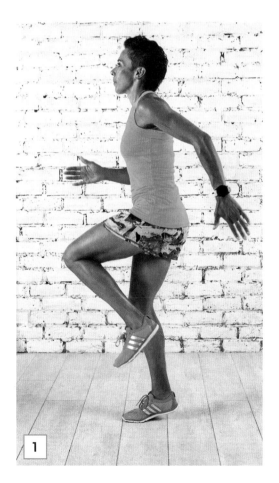

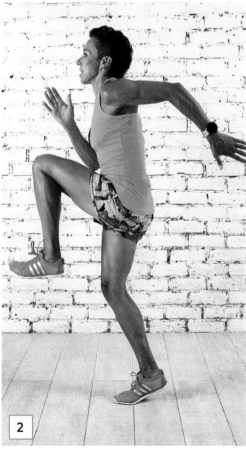

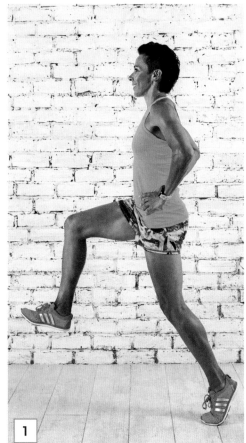

LUNGES

Lunges target the glutes, but involve other muscles, including the quads, hamstrings, calves and core, making them an important exercise for toning the lower body and for stability.

1. Engage the core and keep your body straight and chest lifted.

2. Step forward with your right leg until your front thigh is parallel to the floor, then push your right heel into the ground. Then push back to your starting position with your left leg.

3. Repeat on the opposite side.

4. Perform at least 12 reps on each side to complete one set. Aim for 3 sets.

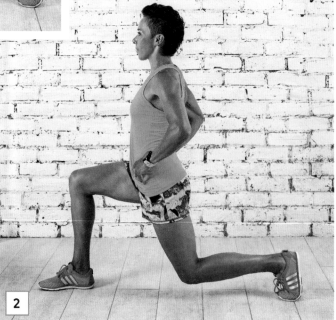

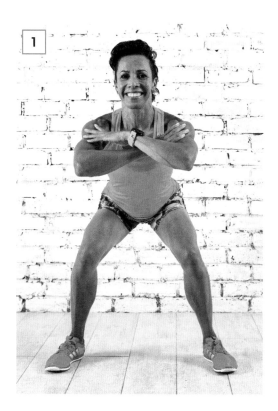

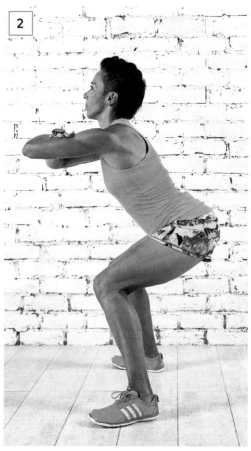

SQUATS

Squats work the quads, hamstrings, glutes and hips all at once. Squats can make you a faster sprinter because they increase your explosive power. They also can make you a faster long-distance runner as leg strength improves endurance. I am not the best at squats and generally need something under my heels to help me sit back.

1. Stand with your feet about shoulder-width apart. Place your hands on the opposite shoulder or position your arms parallel with the ground.

2. Next, while sticking your bum out and folding at the hips, squat down until both knees are bent at a 90-degree angle, and/or both thighs are parallel to the ground. Make sure the back is straight, shoulders and chest upright throughout the movement.

3. Stand back up, driving through the heels. Perform 15–25 reps to complete one set. Repeat three times.

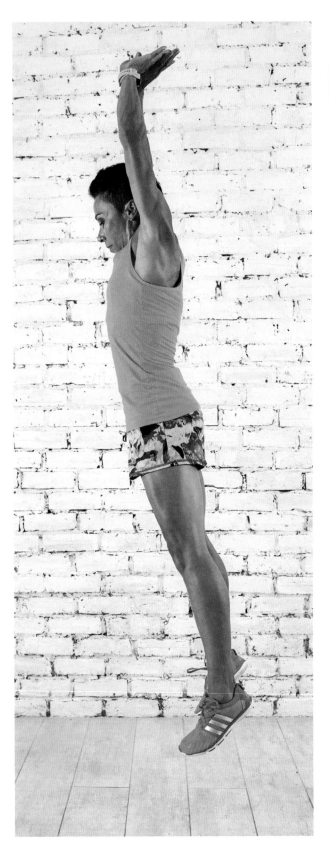

JUMP SQUATS

These increase your explosive power, improve upper- and lower-body strength, and burn calories faster than regular squats. Plus, the flexibility gained in your ankles and hips from the fluid motion of a jump squat will help prevent injuries during other exercise routines.

1. Stand up tall with your feet shoulder-width apart.

2. Start by doing a regular squat (see page 107), then engage your core and jump up explosively.

3. When you land, lower your body back into the squat position to complete one rep. Land as softly as possible, which requires control.

4. Aim for 2–3 sets of 10 reps.

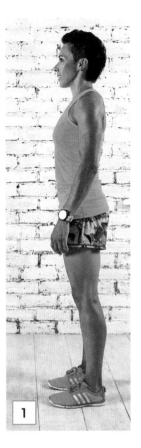

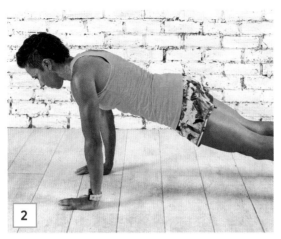

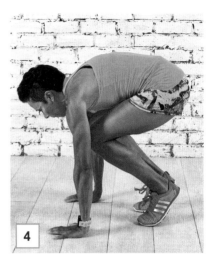

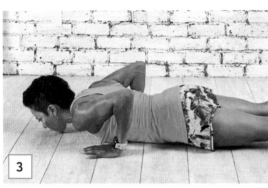

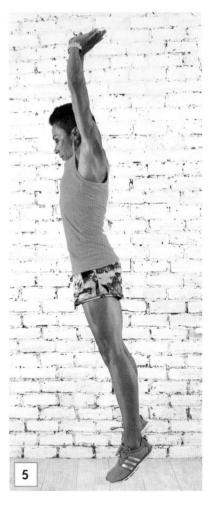

BURPEES

When I was in the army this was definitely the exercise of torture! I was on the giving and receiving end, prescribing them to the soldiers when I was a physical training instructor!

1. From a standing position, squat down and place both hands on the floor in front of you.

2. Jump your feet back into a high plank position.

3. For advanced burpees, go down into a press-up position.

4. Push back up and jump your feet forward.

5. Jump up explosively, raising your hands above your head.

HOME WORKOUTS – STAIRS

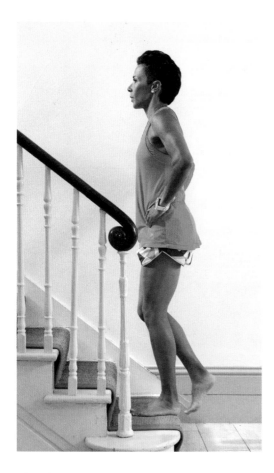

1. Step up onto your step or stair with your right foot driving your left knee high and fully extend your right leg.

2. Step back down with your left foot. Use the opposite arm in a running action so when the arm moves to the front, the hand should come up to the chin. Try 10–25 reps x 2–3 sets.

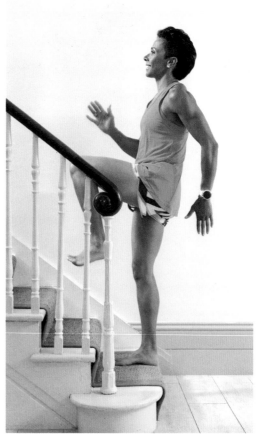

STEP-UPS

1. Find a step or stairs. Step up with one foot, placing it fully on to your platform.

2. Using that leg, lift your body up onto the platform, and end by placing the opposite foot next to your lead foot.

3. Step down with the lead foot, followed by the opposite foot. Alternate your lead leg. Try 10–25 reps x 2–3 sets.

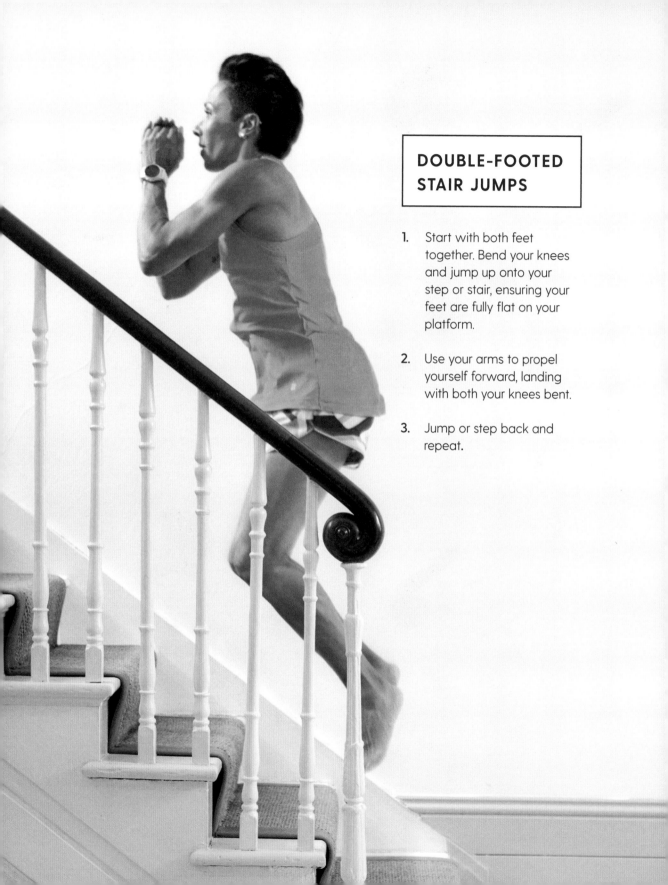

DOUBLE-FOOTED STAIR JUMPS

1. Start with both feet together. Bend your knees and jump up onto your step or stair, ensuring your feet are fully flat on your platform.

2. Use your arms to propel yourself forward, landing with both your knees bent.

3. Jump or step back and repeat.

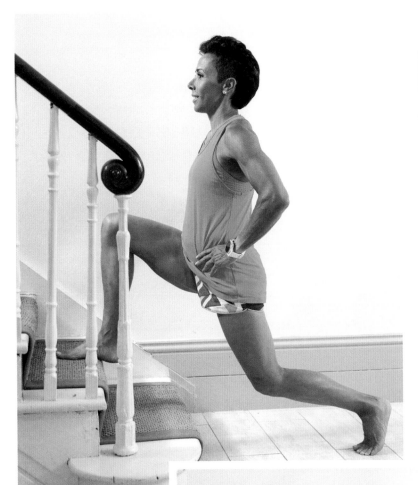

PULSE LUNGES

1. Stand upright facing the step or stairs with one foot on your platform. The toes of both feet should be facing straight ahead.

2. Pulse down and up for 10–15 reps and repeat for 2–3 sets..

3. Repeat on the opposite leg..

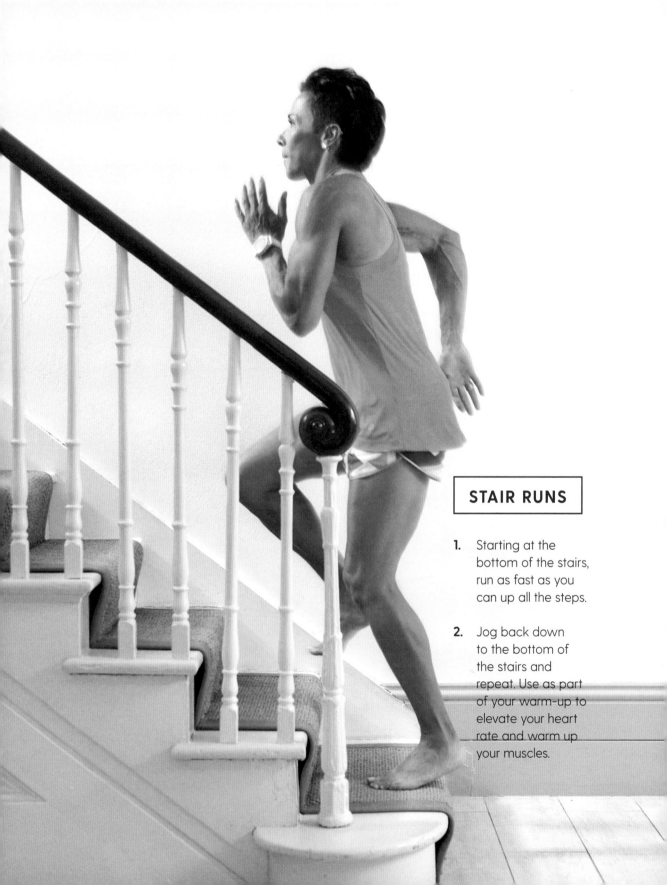

STAIR RUNS

1. Starting at the bottom of the stairs, run as fast as you can up all the steps.

2. Jog back down to the bottom of the stairs and repeat. Use as part of your warm-up to elevate your heart rate and warm up your muscles.

HOME WORKOUTS – BED

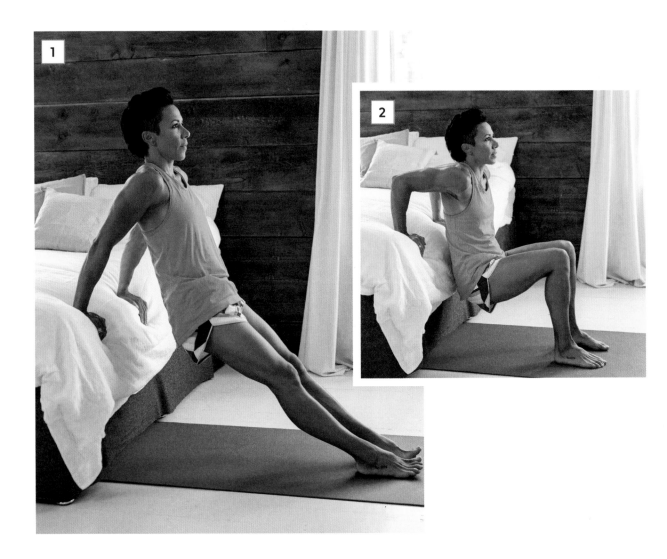

TRICEP DIPS

1. Sit on the bed, place your hands facing forwards and shoulder-width apart. Slide your bum off the edge of the bed with your legs extended in front of you (or for an easier option bend your legs). Straighten your arms, keeping a little bend in your elbows.

2. Lower yourself down so your elbows are at 90 degrees, then push back up to your starting position. Try 10–25 reps x 2–3 sets.

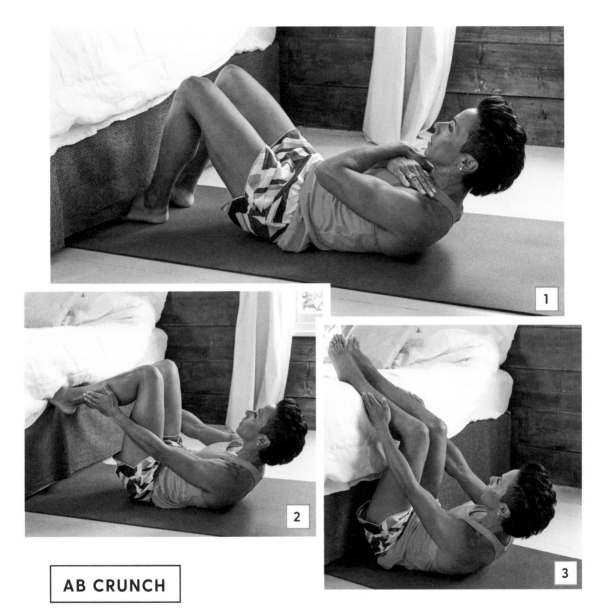

AB CRUNCH

1. Lie on the floor with your feet under the bed. Contract your abs and tighten your core by pulling your belly button towards your spine. Lift your shoulders off the floor then lower back down and repeat.

2. For an intermediate option, bring your feet up to 90 degrees.

3. For an advanced option, bring your bum closer to the bed and lift your legs so that they're almost vertical. Try 10–25 reps x 2–3 sets.

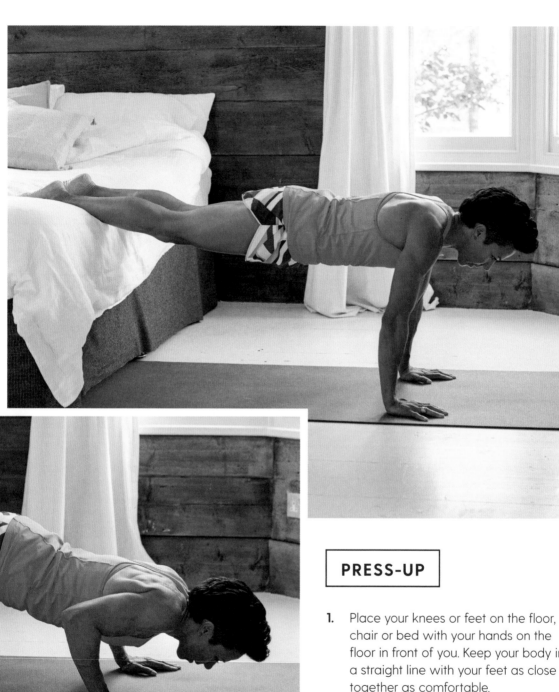

PRESS-UP

1. Place your knees or feet on the floor, chair or bed with your hands on the floor in front of you. Keep your body in a straight line with your feet as close together as comfortable.

2. Bend your elbows to lower your upper body and press back up to the start. Try 10–25 reps x 2–3 sets.

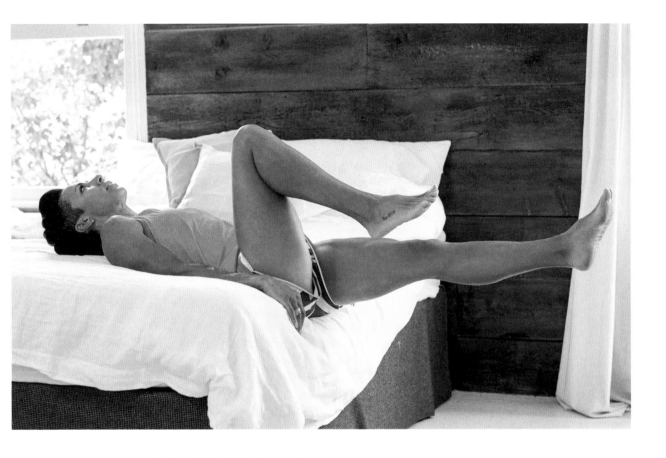

BICYCLE KICKS

1. Lie face up on the floor or a bed with your hands by your sides. Contract your abs and tighten your core by pulling your belly button towards your spine. Keep a tight core throughout the entire exercise.

2. Lift one knee in toward your chest while lifting your shoulder blades off the floor or bed.

3. To take this a step further, bring the opposite elbow towards the knee as you extend the other leg. Alternate each side in a pedalling motion. Try 10–25 reps x 2–3 sets.

JUMP ROPE WORKOUT

These burn loads of calories, improve your foot speed, increase co-ordination and boost agility.

HERE'S AN EXAMPLE WORKOUT ROUTINE:
Start with a 5-minute forward jumping rope exercise at a comfortable pace as a warm-up. Then perform the following exercises:

- `60 seconds of forward jumps`
- `60 seconds of alternate foot jumps`
- `60 seconds of side-to-side jumps`
- `60 seconds of high knees`
- `60 seconds of one-foot hops`
- `60 seconds of double unders (if you're feeling like a boxer!)`

Rest for 1–2 minutes. Repeat the circuit 2–3 times.
Finish the session with a 10-minute cool down.

Other workouts you could do to improve your running:

• PLYOMETRIC

Also known as explosive training, plyometric training requires your muscles to make use of maximum force in minimum time. Running is, in its basic form, an extended series of hops from one leg to the other. With plyometric training, you can isolate and intensify the jumping element in your running, which will boost your running performance without doing more mileage. The plyometric exercises that are a must for runners are the kind of plyo moves that improve push-off power, ankle range of motion, increase stride length and improve overall cardiovascular conditioning.

• BATTLE ROPE TRAINING

Battle ropes are often thought of as exercising for your upper body. However, battle rope workouts also work the muscles in your abs, back and glutes, and you can incorporate movements such as jumps, lunges and squats, that work your legs, too.

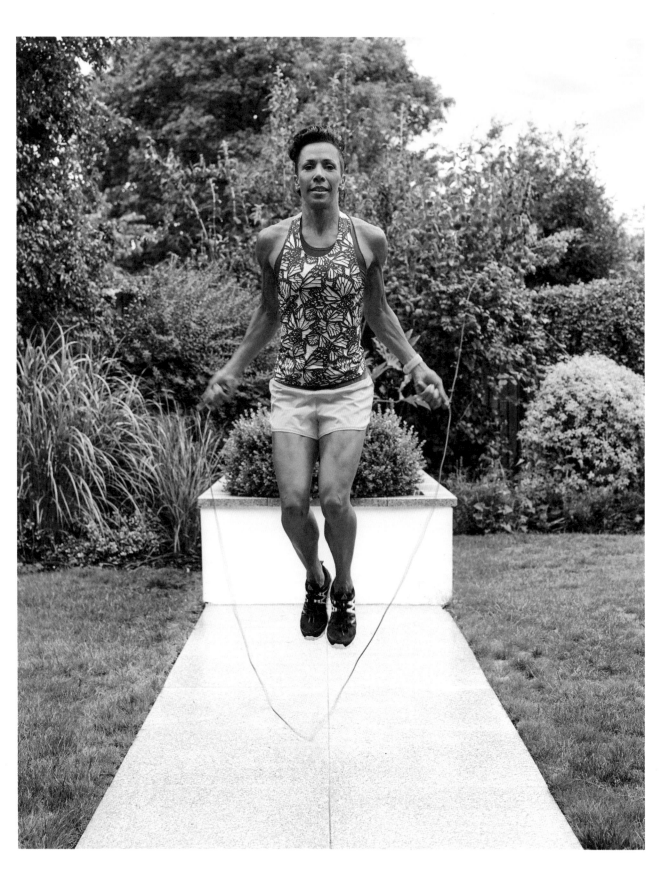

Running isn't just running

Even though I have run all my life, I think it is important to understand that to improve your running you don't just run!

For much of my international career I had to battle through injuries, both mental and physical, learning to adapt my training in order to stay physically fit, motivated and focused on still getting back to running in time for big championships. I don't believe that an injury stops you training, you just have to work around it.

HERE ARE 5 CARDIOVASCULAR CROSS-TRAINING METHODS I USE:

 STEPPER MACHINES
There are two kinds of step machines. A stepper and a stairmaster or stairmill.

• **Stairmaster**
The stairmaster is a favourite cardio choice of mine for a number of reasons. Most importantly, it targets your glutes and thighs and I definitely get a sweat on, plus you can do both high-intensity interval training (HIIT) and low-intensity steady-state cardio (LISS).

The climbing and pushing resistance required to use a stairmaster makes for an excellent lower body workout, which focuses on the calves, glutes, quads, and hamstrings, so you will burn fat and build strength and lean muscle mass.

• **Stepper**
Steppers are a great form of cardiovascular fitness. They simulate climbing flights of stairs, which is a vigorous activity that works the glutes, quads, hamstrings and calf muscles. With a stepper you have to push yourself by increasing the speed to maximise the cardiovascular benefits.

 WATER RUNNING
I am not a water baby, but water running helped me prolong my career and allowed me to stay fit and motivated in order to still win medals.

Water running is more commonly known in the sporting world as aqua jogging because of the AquaJogger® buoyancy belt, which is required for deep water running to ensure good form and posture. This has long been recognised as a rehabilitation exercise for injured athletes, but it's also a great workout.

There are two types of water running: shallow water running, where you run in waist-deep water, across the bottom of the pool, mainly for resistance training or for rehabilitation. And then there is deep water running, where you are in deep enough water that your feet don't touch the bottom of the pool. Any runner looking to increase their cardiovascular capacity without impact and wear and tear on muscles should try deep water running.

As it is non-weight bearing, there is no impact on your body, which allows you to increase your mileage with a lot less risk of injury. You are able to vary the intensity, time or do your favourite fartlek workout (page 93) in the water. It boosts your fitness as well as keeping you focused on getting back to outdoor running.

Heart rates in the water are said to be around 22–25 beats per minute lower than they would be in normal running environments (while performing the same activity at the same intensity level). Researchers say that it is because the water temperature is a bit lower than your own body temperature and water pressure on the body helps circulate your blood, requiring less work from your heart.

A FEW TIPS FOR WATER TRAINING:

- UPPER BODY: Don't lean too far forward. Straighten your upper body, keeping your chest and head up!

- LOWER BODY: You need to bring your knees up more than you would on the road. When you push down, you want a flat foot so you feel as though you're pushing off the water. Then, bring your knee up to about a 90-degree angle. Repeat. And repeat for your session.

- INTENSITY: Work hard! The advantage is you can do a lot and train more regularly without the risks of overtraining.

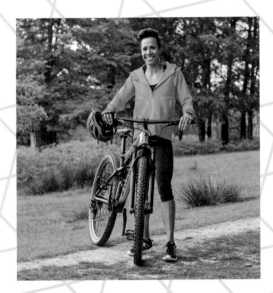 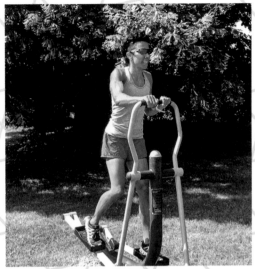

BENEFITS OF CROSS TRAINING

	Low Impact	Upper Body	Lower Body	Core	Full Range
Stepper	✓✓		✓✓✓	✓✓	✓
Water Running	✓✓✓	✓✓✓	✓✓✓✓	✓✓	✓✓✓
Cross Trainer/ Elliptical	✓✓✓	✓✓	✓✓✓	✓✓	✓✓
Cycling	✓✓✓	✓	✓✓✓	✓	✓✓✓
Rower	✓✓✓	✓✓✓	✓✓✓	✓✓✓	✓✓✓

3 CROSS TRAINER/ELLIPTICAL

The great advantage of a cross trainer, or an elliptical, is that it allows you to work both upper body muscles (biceps, triceps, abs, pectorals) and the lower body (glutes, hamstrings, quads and calves). To maximise the effect of an elliptical, pedal backwards using your glutes and hamstrings, bend at the hips a little as though you're going to sit down, while keeping your knees at a 90-degree angle as you stride.

It helps you work your cardiovascular system and heart, can improve your endurance and maintain your fitness, burns calories and therefore can help you to lose weight while toning your muscles.

4 INDOOR OR OUTDOOR CYCLING

Indoor cycling is a low-impact activity and is good whether you are recovering from injury or not, as it avoids stress on your joints.

When you are pedalling against resistance, you increase the endurance of the leg muscles. Working these muscles also helps to strengthen surrounding bones, tendons and ligaments, increasing overall strength. We've all heard about the runner's high. An indoor cycling class can provide that same rush of adrenaline and a release of happy-mood endorphins. It can also keep your heart rate at an intense range for a continuous period to improve fitness.

I also love cycling on or off-road, which works various muscles to increase strength and flexibility and improve posture and co-ordination.

5 ROWING MACHINE

The rowing machine is fantastic for working out your whole body. Both your upper and lower body are required to complete a full rowing stroke, and therefore nearly every muscle is used.

You get a solid workout that's guaranteed to get you sweating. Through every phase you are working quads, hamstrings, glutes, lats, core, shoulders, triceps, back and biceps as well as of lots of smaller muscles. The rowing machine effectively raises your heart rate and provides an excellent overall aerobic workout, making this a fantastic training machine for fitness and muscle endurance.

MY FAVOURITE EIGHT RECOVERY TECHNIQUES

1. Recovery runs

HOW DO YOU KNOW IF YOU ARE DOING YOUR RECOVERY RUNS RIGHT? BASICALLY THEY SHOULD FEEL EASY!

A   Run at a pace where you can sustain a conversation, as this means you are working aerobically, but not going anywhere near oxygen debt. If you use a heart rate monitor, this may be around of 50–60% of your maximum heart rate.

B   Choose a softer surface like grass, trails or tracks. As recovery runs are a slower speed, they are also at a low percentage of a runner's maximum oxygen uptake.

C   Focus on your running technique, as you should be going easy enough to be able to pay attention to exactly how you are running.

2. Stretching/mobility

A   Studies have shown that regularly performing static stretching can help to decrease stiffness and reduce any aches or pains (especially in individuals with chronic neck or low-back pain).

B   Various types of stretching (as well as other supportive self-care strategies such as self-myofascial releasing using a foam roller) can help to enhance movement of the major joints, including key areas that are designed to be mobile, such as the hips and shoulders.

C   Dynamic stretches/mobility exercises are often used as part of a warm-up to help increase core body temperature and prepare the body for the movements that are to come. Stretching can help enhance agility, power, speed and muscular strength.

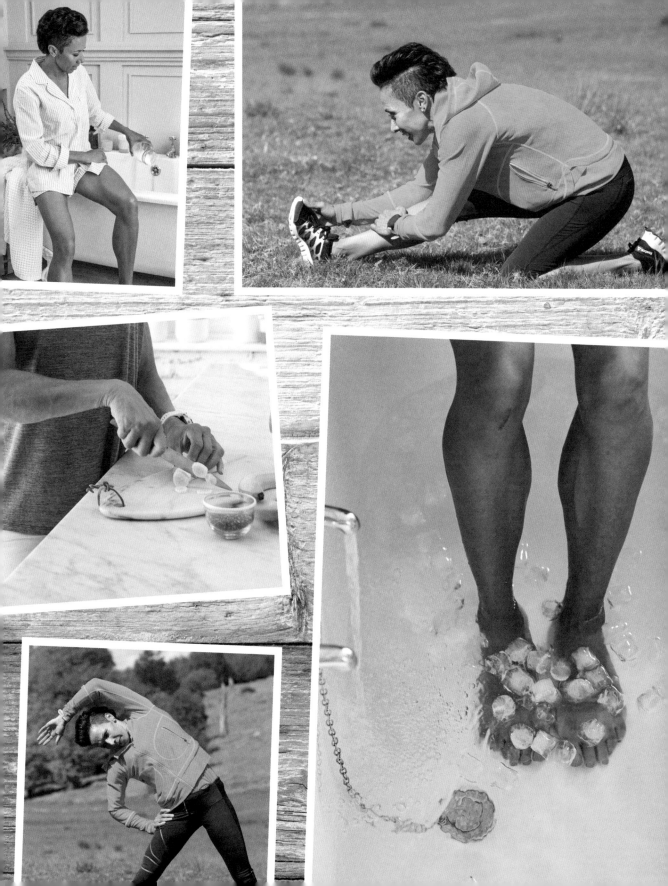

3. Epsom salts

A   Appropriate levels of magnesium are absolutely key to good health, and it is common to have a magnesium deficiency. Soak your feet or entire body in a bath containing Epsom salts to naturally increase internal levels of magnesium without taking supplements.

B   **REDUCES STRESS** – Everyone has heard of the recommendation to have a good soak in a warm bath after a rough day (whether mentally or physically) as it's a great way to bust stress. If you want to amplify the stress-reducing benefits of a nice long soak, add a cup or two of Epsom salts to your bathwater. Not only will the magnesium in the Epsom salts help to relax your muscles, it can also help to relax your mind.

C   **REDUCES TOXINS** – The sulfates in Epsom salts assist the body in flushing out toxins and provide a detox for the body's cells, lowering the internal accumulation of harmful substances. Adding minerals like magnesium and sulfate to your bath sparks a process called reverse osmosis, which pulls salts and toxins out of your body.

D   **REDUCES PAIN & INFLAMMATION** – A warm bath containing Epsom salts is known to ease pain and relieve inflammation, making it beneficial for sore muscles. Epsom salts can also help reduce the swelling that accompanies sprains and bruises.

E   **IMPROVES BLOOD SUGAR LEVELS** – Magnesium and sulfate help improve the body's ability to produce and utilise insulin. Regular intake of Epsom salts through the skin can help to regulate blood sugar, lowering the risk of diabetes and improving daily energy levels.

FOR A DETOXIFYING BATH

Add at least 2 cups of Epsom salts to bathwater and soak for 40 minutes. The first 20 minutes will help to remove toxins while the last twenty will allow you to absorb the minerals and emerge feeling rejuvenated. Consume water before, during and after to prevent dehydration and increase detoxification.

4. Ice baths

I used to have a lot of these when I was competing; I hate ice and cold water and it takes me longer to get in them than to actually be submersed, but they are totally worthwhile.

A   Known as cold water immersion or cryotherapy, it is a method to reduce swelling and recovery time after a hard session. It is used to recover faster and reduce muscle pain and soreness after intense training sessions or competitions. In addition to the ice bath, some athletes use contrast water therapy (alternating between cold water and warmer water) to get the same effect or more like a flush effect.

B   With any sprain, strain or bruise there is some bleeding into the underlying tissues. This causes swelling and pain. Ice treatment may be used in both the immediate treatment of soft tissue injuries and in later rehabilitation. They can reduce pain by numbing the area and by limiting swelling.

5. Bananas

There are a handful of foods that may assist recovery. Bananas contain potassium, a mineral that is crucial to heart function and muscle contraction. People who have low potassium levels may experience muscle soreness and cramping.

6. Protein

Dietary protein is required to promote growth, repair damaged cells and tissues, synthesise hormones, and for a variety of metabolic activities. There are multiple sources of protein, however, animal protein contains all essential amino acids and is considered a complete source of protein, whereas plant protein lacks some of the essential amino acids and is therefore 'incomplete'. There is significant evidence that people doing intense training require more dietary protein (1.4–2g/kg body weight a day). For most people, this can be obtained from a regular and varied diet. However, recent evidence indicates that ingesting protein and/or amino acids prior to, during and/or following exercise can enhance recovery, immune function and growth and maintenance of lean body mass.

7. Hydration

A   Drinking water after a tough workout can help rid your body of toxins and prevent dehydration.

B   We need 2–3 litres a day to transport nutrients, to help with digestion, to carry out waste and toxins and to support brain function for mood, energy and concentration.

C   We lose water and body salts (mostly sodium and chloride) through urine but also when we sweat. Even more fluids are lost during exercise, and a water loss of only 1–2% of our body weight can impair performance by 10–20%!

To prevent dehydration, increase this amount if you're exercising. Sports drinks which contain carbohydrate (CHO) in the form of glucose can help replenish glycogen stores to boost energy. Equally, don't over-drink. When sodium levels are depleted to dangerous levels, which then dilutes the concentration of sodium in the blood, it can result in confusion and lack of co-ordination. Although it takes quite a lot of water to get to this point, it's good to be aware of it, especially if you are training for a long endurance event like a marathon.

```
WHEN TO HYDRATE

•  Exercise under 30 minutes
No need to drink while exercising (unless it's very
warm), but rehydrate with water afterwards.

•  Exercise from 30-60 minutes
As above, then rehydrate post-training with a
drink containing both water and carbohydrate.

•  Exercise 1-3 hours
Take a sports drink with you that combines
water, electrolytes and CHO. Sip throughout
the session - aim for 30-60g CHO per hour.
Continue to use the same drink post-training.
```

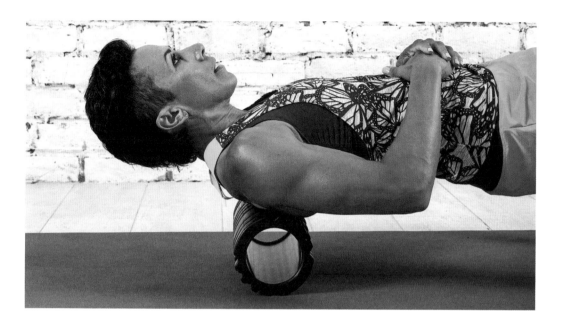

8. Massage/foam rolling

A   Sports massage is for managing, manipulating and rehabilitating soft tissues throughout the body. One of the main aims of a sports massage is to relieve tightness/tension. I can't tell you how much they have helped me both with recovery and prevention of problems.

B   A sports massage will stretch and lengthen your muscles in a much deeper and more specific way than when you stretch after your run.

C   Blood flow to a particular area is increased and improved, meaning that healing can take place and so the muscles are rejuvenated.

D   It increases flexibility to improve your range of motion and joint mobility. This can reduce the chance of injury occurring or reoccurring.

E   Breaking down scar tissue. Massage will help to break down scar tissue, promoting correct, strong scar formation in the muscle.

F   It can also help with the removal of lactic acid and other waste products caused by slight tears in or overuse of the muscle.

G   Foam rolling is a self-help tool and, much like massage, helps reduce tightness and increases blood flow. Slow movements help to break down scar tissue and speed up healing and recovery.

case studies

Kelly asked me to look at her running technique for this book. I have known Kelly for many years as her physio, but this is how I would look at her if she came to see me now, both as a patient and as an athlete looking to improve their running technique.

Kelly's technique is by and large a textbook classic for a runner. I wouldn't be looking to change much, but there are a few things that could be addressed to help Kelly be more efficient and resilient. As an athlete, she was getting physio on a very regular basis, as the focus was on keeping her in one piece and allowing her to be able to train and race at the highest level.

Kelly's leg function is good at steady state and tempo pace. She lands with the foot underneath the body and lands between the forefoot and midfoot. There is no cross over of the midline of the body.

Kelly has limited ankle range due to soft tissue tightness through the calves and feet, and she also has stiff joints in the ankles and feet. This is something we worked on every week in the two years before the 2004 Olympics to allow Kelly to have optimal foot function. If Kelly was seeing a physio regularly, this is something that would ideally be treated each time. She would also be given a lot of self-help work to do to maintain this.

Kelly is very strong and stable, which is a testament to the type of training that she does. This is the main reason that she has been able to train at the level and speed she has. Kelly has also done drills and technique work for years and years to run as technically well as she does.

The main area in which Kelly could improve is through the torso, hips and pelvis. To run most efficiently, the rib cage should be able to counter-rotate on the pelvis. Counter-rotation is the ability for the two parts of the body to rotate in opposite directions. There should also be sufficient mobility at the hips, so that there is minimal effect of moving the legs on the pelvis. Looking at video footage of Kelly running, she tends to side flex through the trunk rather than having the subtle rotation that would be more efficient. Increased side flexion of the trunk will tend to make the hips and feet overwork, as they have to compensate for the extra movement and for balance, as the central axis of the body is not falling over the pelvis in the same way. Kelly is quite stiff in rotation through the upper body, in part due to muscle tightness through the upper back and in part due to tightness in the abdomen. I would do some soft tissue work to the muscles around the spine and rib cage, and some joint mobilisation work. I would then also suggest that she does

EXERCISE

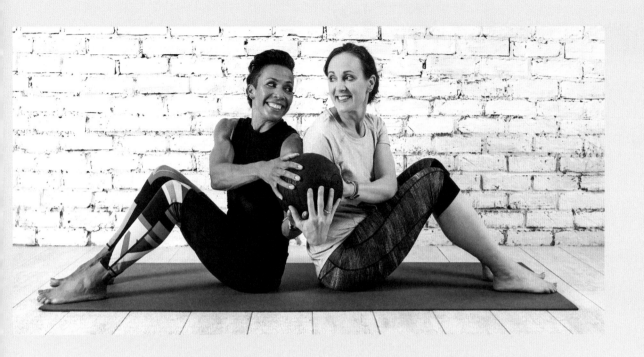

exercises to retrain how the torso and pelvis counter-rotate on each other, which may be rotation of the trunk in sitting, lunges with rotation, or drills and balance work involving rotation (see pages 136–149). Kelly is also very tight in the muscles in the hips and glutes, and she also has some limited extension at the hips, due in part to the hip flexors being short, and I would look at increasing mobility through these areas as well.

Kelly tends to 'flick' her right leg when running at speed on the bend of the track, especially as she tires (so she is a Flicker, see pages 134–135) – I suspect that this is due to not having sufficient soft tissue length through the trunk and hip flexors. As she rotates to the left, on a bend, with the right leg in extension, she then needs to flick the leg around to bring it through. This could be improved with the treatment described above. Kelly also complains of having a tired and heavy feeling in the right leg, which gives her a feeling of dragging when she is running up hills. This is probably due to the same issues, which will have an effect on muscle function and efficiency.

There are a few areas that Kelly could address to help her become more robust, more efficient, to be more comfortable when running and to help her run more often. It would definitely be worth looking at this, to help Kelly run for many years to come while minimising the risk of injury.

run better

I AM VERY AWARE THAT DURING MY ATHLETICS CAREER IT WAS THE STORY OF MY FIGHT BACK THAT DOMINATED THE SPORTS NEWS, RATHER THAN MY ACTUAL ATHLETICS CREDENTIALS.

Achilles tendons and calf muscle injuries were the bane of my life. When you are at the level I was, there is always a fine line between being on top form – strong, fit, focused – and being injured – weak in body and mind. It was a case of managing my injuries rather than preventing them, because the level I was running at was so intense, I was pushing my body to its very limits.

Towards the end of my career I had a great support team when it came to managing my injuries, especially Alison Rose, a chartered physiotherapist and clinical director/owner of The Coach House Sports Physiotherapy Clinic in Leeds. While writing this book, we were discussing how techniques have changed and how she wishes that she knew back then what she knows now. Having had serious setbacks that threatened my career on numerous occasions, sometimes it could all seem doom and gloom. But it is testament to my team's perseverance and their professionalism, as well my ability to believe in myself, that we got to the top of the Olympic podium.

At an elite level I was fortunate to have medical care and access to some great doctors, physiotherapists, nutritionists, surgeons and sports scientists but I know too well that most people do not. If you are able to afford it, do try to consult a physiotherapist to ensure you are given appropriate advice.

Running can be difficult enough when you are training to get better, but not being efficient can make it a whole lot harder. This got me thinking about how I could help you to identify your running style so that you can get the most out of your running, perform at your very best and enjoy what you do, however you do it. This section will enable you to identify your running style, understand the problem, see the solution and do exercises that will help you strengthen and stabilise weak areas in order to enhance your running.

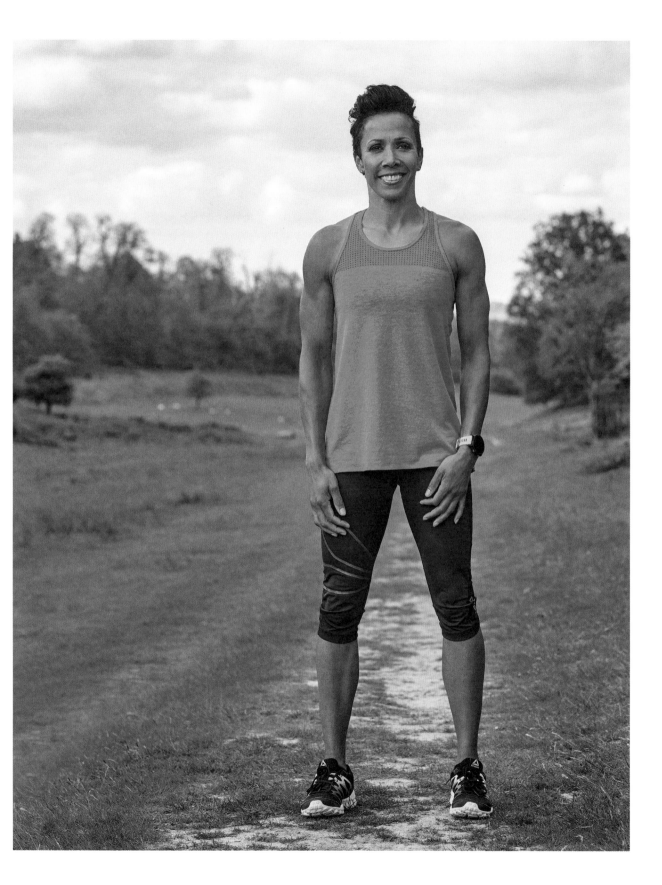

Are you a flicker or a flapper?

	problem	solution	exercise
FLICKER	Legs flicking out from knee, tend to have poor foot placement and reduced glute strength.	Improve hip movement pattern Increase range length of TFL Assess glute and abductor strength Assess hamstring strength Adductor length	Calf stretches (page 136) Squats (page 137) One-leg standing (page 137) Golf ball rolls (page 144) Hip circles (page 141) Abductor strength (page 147)
DRIVER	Mid foot runner – strikes ground midway between the ball and heel of foot, need to make sure there is enough mobility in the foot and calf to do this safely.	Improve calf strength and length, and ankle mobility to enable safer mid-foot strike and better roll through and push off ankle. Improve foot mobility	Squats (page 137) One-leg standing (page 137) Hip circles (page 141) Lunges (page 144) Golf ball rolls (page 144)
HUNCHER/ SWINGER	Rounded upper back with shoulders forward, quite often poor in thoracic counter rotation.	Stretch anterior muscles from neck to front of thigh (quads). Postural work Movement pattern retraining Spinal stability Thoracic mobillity	One-leg standing (page 137) 4-point kneeling and Swiss ball steering wheels (page 139) Alternate knee drives (page 145) Straight leg calf raises (page 145)
SCUFFLER	No knee lift, limited hip movement and no stride length. Poor use of calves.	Strengthen and improve lower limb mobility, especially in the hips. Improve movement patterning of the hip joint and improve calf strength.	Squats (page 137) Step up into drive (page 138) Hip circles (page 141) Lunges (page 144) Straight leg calf raises (page 145) Bridge (page 148)
KNEE KNOCKER	Knees fall in towards midline of body.	Re-educate hip movement pattern Stretch adductors and calves Strengthen abductors Strengthen glute max and external rotators	One-leg standing (page 137) Step up into drive (page 138) Clam (page 140) Hip circles (page 141) Adductor stretch (page 142) Abductor strength (page 147)
SADDLE SITTER	Sitting back with hips tilting backwards, usually tight anterior chest muscles, short hamstrings and weak inner glutes.	Stabilise and improve chest expansion Lots of hip strength, retraining and centring exercises Need to improve hamstring length and glute strength.	Anterior chest stretch (page 138) Squats (page 137) Hip circles (page 141) Adductor stretch (page 142) Counter rotation (page 143) Lunges (page 144)
STICKY PITTER	Arms straight with limited swinging movement – will usually have poor thoracic movment as well to counterbalance lack of movement from the shoulders.	Improve positioning and movment of arms from the shoulders. Awareness of arm position Standing/dynamic balance training	One-leg standing (page 137) Step up into drive (page 138) Counter rotation (page 143) Lunges (page 144) Alternate knee drives (page 145) Hip slapping (page 146)

	problem	*solution*	*exercise*
FLAPPER	Elbow and forearm splaying out.	Stretches – pecs, anterior and shoulder Lots of practise of the correct movement, especially in balance positions.	Anterior chest stretch (page 138) 4-point kneeling and Swiss ball steering wheels (page 139) Alternate knee drives (page 145) Holding item (page 148)
BOUNDER	Exaggerated stride length, tends to over-use quads and hip flexors to lift and drive legs forward.	Improve hip movement pattern, so reducing overuse of muscles anteriorly and increasing use of glutes. Increase calf strength to enable better use of the feet. Encourage shorter stride.	Calf stretches (page 136) Straight leg calf raises (page 145) When running, try to run with slightly shorter strides.
CROSS-OVER	One or both feet cross midline of your body. This will increase load going through the foot and increase the speed of pronation in the foot.	Improve the movement of the femur and the leg and foot to come through in line with the hip. Improve abductor strength and balance.	One-leg standing (page 137) Hip circles (page 141) Straight leg calf raises (page 145) Abductor strength (page 147)
FLOATER	Someone that glides when running – good style.	Pay attention to any areas that may get injured so work on the non-negotiables of calf strength, dynamic balance and lunges.	Calf stretches (page 136) One-leg standing (page 137) Straight leg calf raises (page 145)
HUGGER	Elbow bent with arms close to body and limited swing from the shoulder, usually in response to poor habits or reduced stability; technique will not flow as well as it could.	Stretch anterior chest and pecs Balance work, encourage arm movements and thorax mobility.	One-leg standing (page 137) Anterior chest stretch (page 138) Counter rotation (page 143) Lunges (page 144) Alternate knee drives (page 145)
PRANCER	Forefoot runner – strikes ground on ball of foot as if wearing high heels. Will often have tight quads, hip flexors, and calves.	Improve foot placement and calf length. Improve quad and hip flexor length	Calf stretches (page 136) Hip circles (page 141) Hip flexor stretch (page 142) Straight leg calf raises (page 145)
HEAD BANGER	Head nods forward, usually in response to poor upper body strength, stability and mobility.	Improve pec length, posterior neck strength and balance. Lots of practice of correct head position for all exercises, especially in balance positions.	One-leg standing (page 137) Anterior chest stretch (page 138) 4-point kneeling and Swiss ball steering wheels (page 139) Alternate knee drives (page 145) High knee lifts (page 149)
ROAD KISSER	Leans forward as if about to over balance. Usually lack of awareness of trunk position. Will reduce the activation of the glutes, and affect breathing.	Improve postural awareness, and upper body stability. Improve arm swing. Improve hip function, mobility and stability.	One-leg standing (page 137) Counter rotation (page 143) Lunges (page 144) Alternate knee drives (page 145) High knee lifts (page 149)

run better EXERCISES

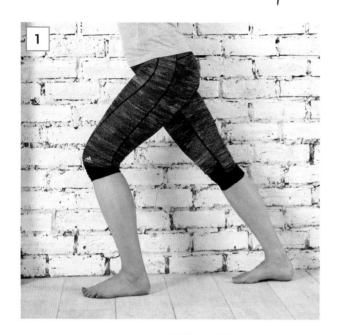

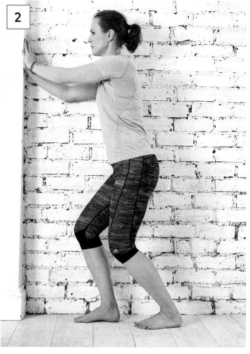

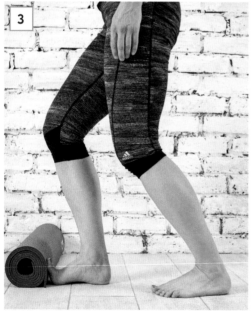

CALF STRETCHES

1. Step one leg forward, keeping both feet flat. Extend the opposite leg straight back with your heel flat. Lean into the wall until you feel the stretch in the bigger calf muscle of the straight leg called the gastrocnemius.

2. Take a half step forward. Keep your weight evenly distributed and slowly bend both knees. You will feel a stretch in the smaller calf muscle above the heel in the back leg called the soleus.

3. Repeat steps 1–2 but press your toes against a rolled up yoga mat for a deeper stretch.

SQUATS

1. Stand with your feet about shoulder-width apart, place your hands on your hips or stretch your arms out straight so they are parallel with the ground.

2. Follow the instructions for Squats on page 107, keeping your hands on your hips or your arms straight out in front of you.

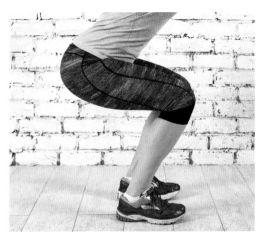

ONE-LEG STANDING

1. Stand tall with your hands by your sides. Keep your toes and arms relaxed.

2. Lift one leg off the floor so you are balancing on the opposite leg. Hold for 30 seconds.

3. For an advanced option, turn your head left and right.

4. Repeat on the opposite leg.

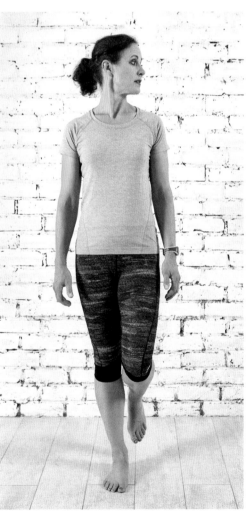

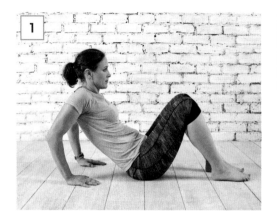

1

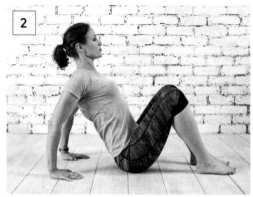

2

ANTERIOR CHEST STRETCH

1. This stretch helps to open out the front of the shoulders to improve posture. Sit on the floor with your knees bent and supporting your torso on your hands.

2. Press through your hands to lift your chest away from the floor until you feel a stretch in the front of your shoulders. Inhale deeply for a count of five to increase the stretch.

STEP UP INTO DRIVE

1. Stand in front of a box or chair and lift one knee to hip height. Drive up and forward through the toes of your standing leg until the front foot lands on the chair. You should be able to maintain posture and feel this in the calf and buttock.

2. Repeat 3 sets of up to 10 reps, focusing on your technique.

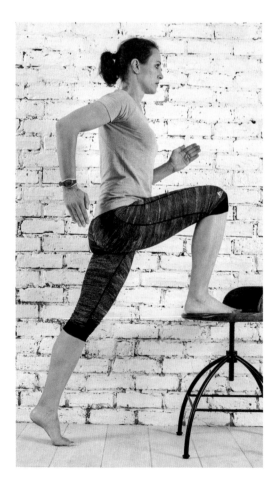

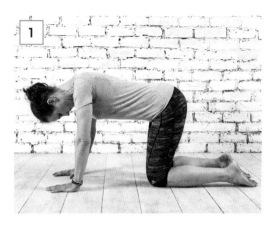

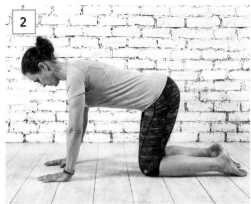

4-POINT KNEELING

1. Start on your hands and knees, with your hands directly under your shoulders and knees directly under your hips. Let your head hang towards the floor and elongate your neck.

2. Lift your neck towards the ceiling until your head and neck are in line with the rest of your spine. Hold this position for up to 10 secs and perform 10 reps.

SWISS BALL STEERING WHEELS

1. This stretch is good for encouraging the shoulder blades to move independently from the thorax as well as thorax stability. Sit on a chair with good posture and hold the Swiss ball in front of you. Maintain your posture while you rotate the Swiss ball like a steering wheel for 10 reps in each direction.

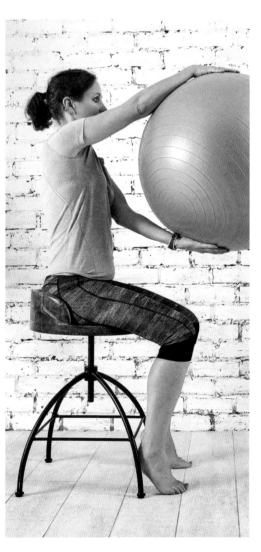

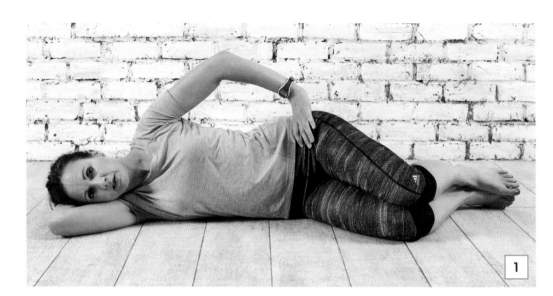

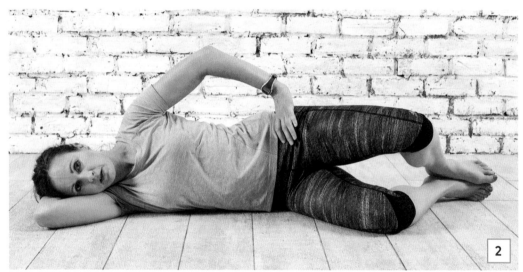

CLAM

1. Lie on your side with your hips and knees bent at a 45-degree angle and the soles of your feet in line with your spine. Lengthen through your waist so there is a small gap between your waist and the floor.

2. Keeping the front of your thigh relaxed, lift the top knee and then lower. You should feel this in your top buttock. Repeat for 30 secs.

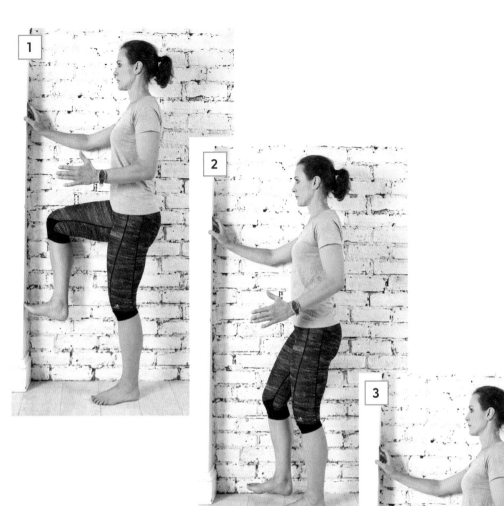

HIP CIRCLES

1. Stand on your left leg with your
    fingertips on a wall and flex the right hip.

2. Bring your right foot back to the floor.
    Circle your right thigh from the hip,
    keeping your back relaxed. Your toes
    should brush close to the wall, but not
    touch it. Perform for 30 seconds, then
    repeat on the opposite leg.

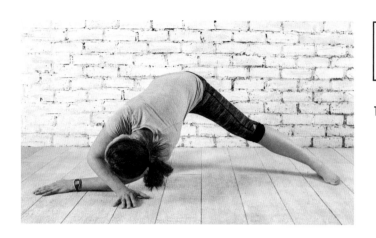

ADDUCTOR STRETCH

1. Start on your hands
    and knees, with your
    hands under your
    shoulders and your
    knees under your hips.
    Take your left leg out to
    the side with your foot
    flat on the floor. Slide
    your left hand under
    your right shoulder until
    you can feel a stretch
    in the left side of your
    ribcage and left inner
    thigh. Breathe for
    5 seconds and repeat
    on the opposite side.

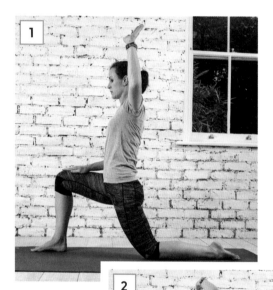

HIP FLEXOR STRETCH

1. Start in a lunge with
    your left knee on the
    floor. Take your weight
    forward onto your right
    leg. Put your right hand
    on top of the right
    leg with your elbow
    at 90 degrees.

2. Side flex towards the
    right (ie towards the
    front leg).

3. Rotate back to the
    other side. Hold for
    30 seconds x 3 reps.

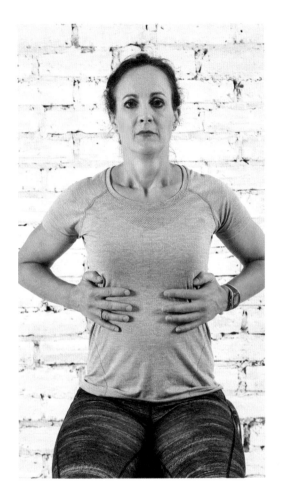

BREATHING

1. Sitting on a chair or stool, place your hands on your lower ribs. Inhale, and feel this area of your rib cage expand laterally as you do so. The movement should not come from the upper ribs at the beginning of the breath. It is good to practise this in front of a mirror, before integrating the movement into your other exercises.

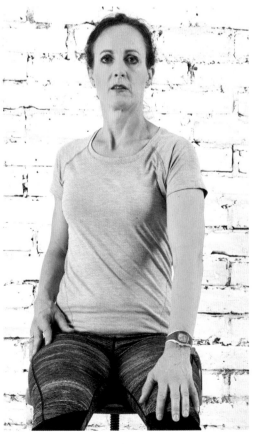

COUNTER ROTATION

1. Sit on a chair or stool with your feet on the floor, with a relaxed posture and your hands on your lap.

2. Keep your head still and rotate through your lower rib cage. Your shoulders will move as your ribs move, they shouldn't be pulling you into rotation. Repeat 20 times.

RUNNING LIFE

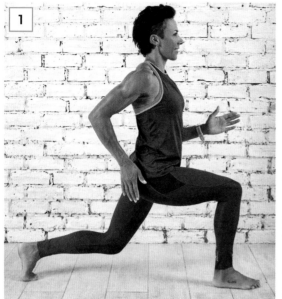

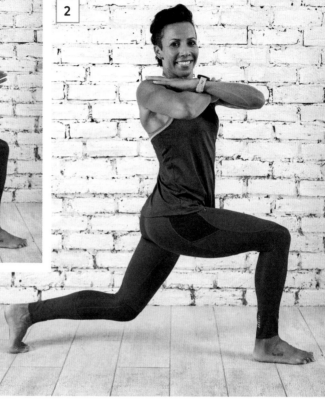

LUNGES

1. Stand with one foot in front of the other, with good posture, the pelvis level and with both hips pointing forwards. Go into a lunge by bending the back knee and relaxing the front buttock to let the front hip fold. Lower the pelvis straight down until the front knee is at 90 degrees.

2. For an advanced option, rotate your waist toward your front leg. Return to the starting position by pushing the front heel down into the floor.

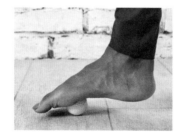

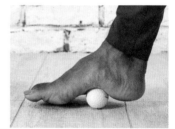

GOLF BALL ROLLS

1. Use a golf or tennis ball to sink into the sole of the foot just in front of the heel and roll the ball towards the toes and back. Sink gently and allow the muscles to relax. Repeat for a maximum of 3 minutes 2-3 times a week.

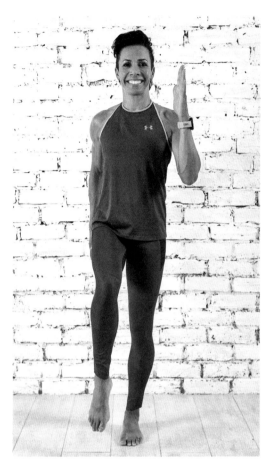

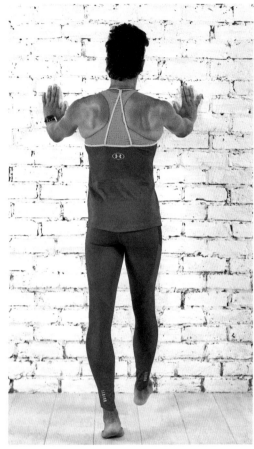

ALTERNATE KNEE DRIVES

1. Standing tall with your chest up, back straight and chin level, swing your arms smoothly and with control, with your hands coming forward to chin level and back to just past your hips. Alternate swinging your legs and bringing the knees up in line with your hips, keeping your foot and toes upwards. Emphasise the driving action (extension) of the support leg at the ankle, knee and hip while stressing a 'tall on your toes' action with the supporting foot.

STRAIGHT LEG CALF RAISES

1. Stand on one leg with your knee straight and your fingers on a wall for balance.

2. Lift the heel of your raised foot up and down, going onto the toes, keeping the knee straight and lifting the heel as high as you can. Build up to 3 sets of 25 reps and perform after running.

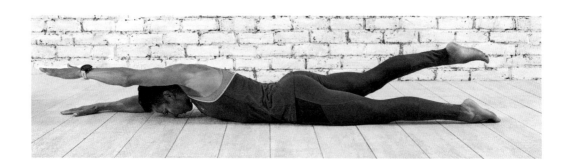

SUPERMAN

1. Lie on the floor on your stomach and draw your stomach muscles up from the floor.

2. Lift your left arm and right leg off the floor, without hyperextending the back. Hold for a count of 5 seconds and perform 5 reps on each side.

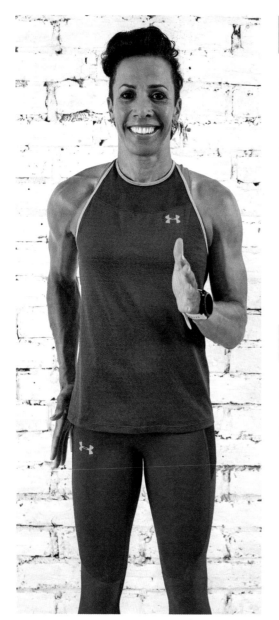

HIP SLAPPING

1. Stand tall with your knees slightly bent.

2. Your shoulders should be relaxed and allow your arms to swing with little effort. Your elbows should be at a 90-degree angle. Your arms should swing alongside the torso with your elbows able to come behind you and your hands slapping your hips. This helps improve your running and prevent your arms coming across your body.

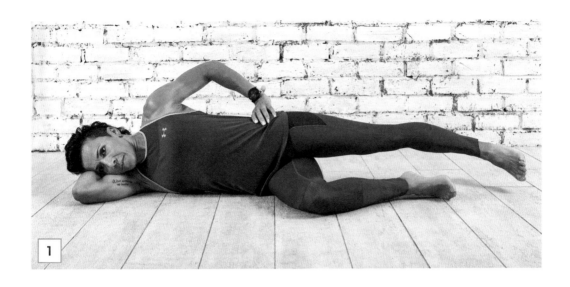

ABDUCTOR STRENGTH

1. Lie on your side with your bottom knee bent and your top leg straight and far enough back so you can't see your top knee.

2. Raise and lower your top leg to hip height from the *hip joint only*. Repeat for 30 seconds x 2 sets with your toes pointing forward and your knee behind your hip.

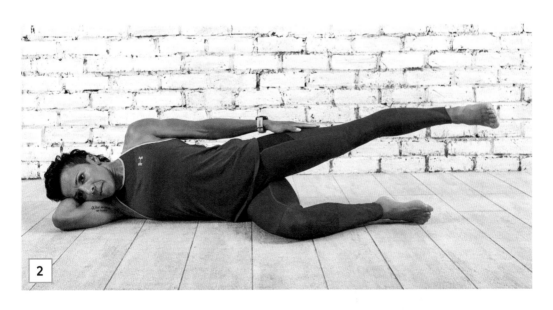

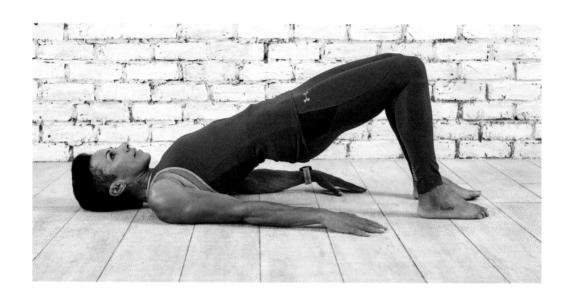

BRIDGE

1. Lie on your back and start to activate your abs. Keep your lower back flat against the floor. Bend your knees at a 90-degree angle with your feet flat Your arms can just rest right by your side, palms facing down.

2. Lift your hips and engage your glutes. Push your feet into the floor as you lift your hips. Hold.

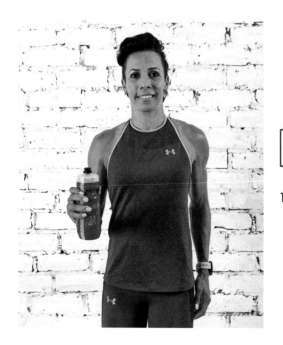

HOLDING ITEM

1. This exercise can help you to improve your arm swing. Simply hold something in your hands while you are doing drills, other exercises or running. If you feel this doesn't help, this is not appropriate for you.

HIGH KNEE LIFTS

1. Keeping your right leg straight, draw your left heel up under your buttock and your knee in front of your pelvis. Repeat on the spot with the same leg, bringing in running arm movements.

2. To make it more dynamic, this drill can be done by alternating the support foot and the working foot.

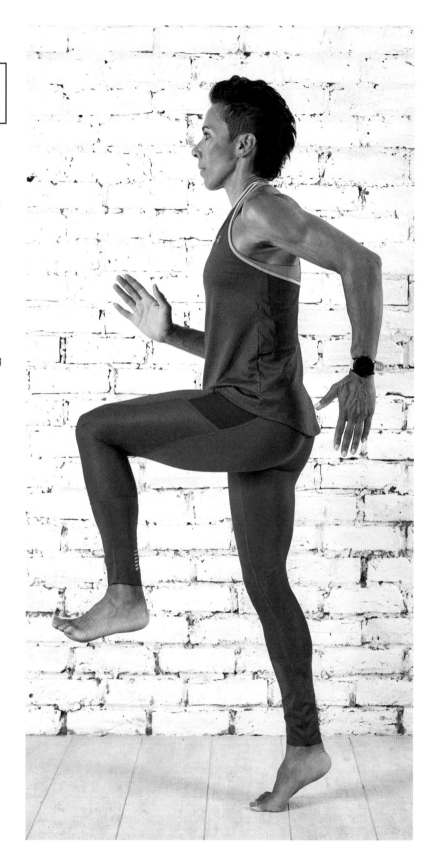

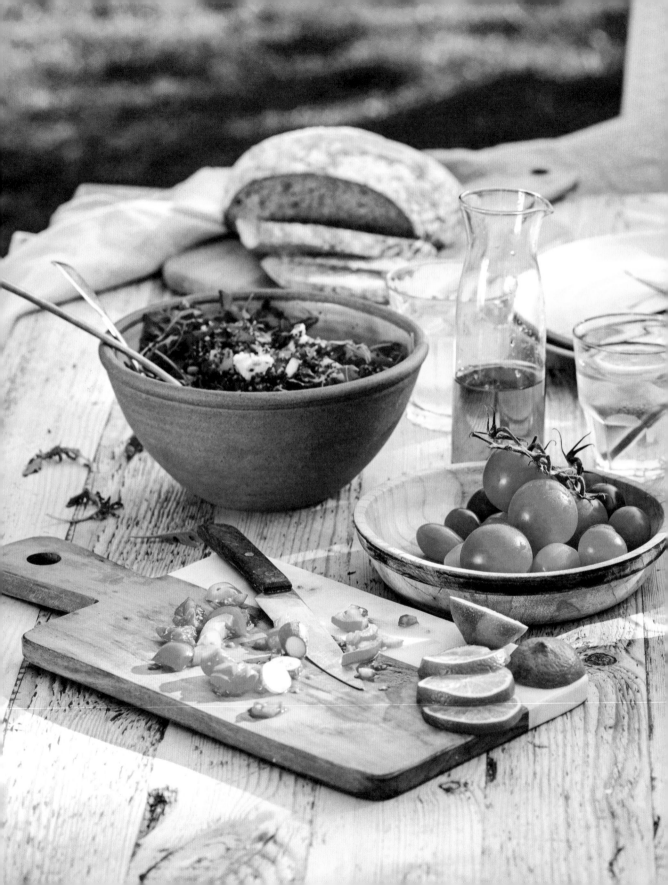

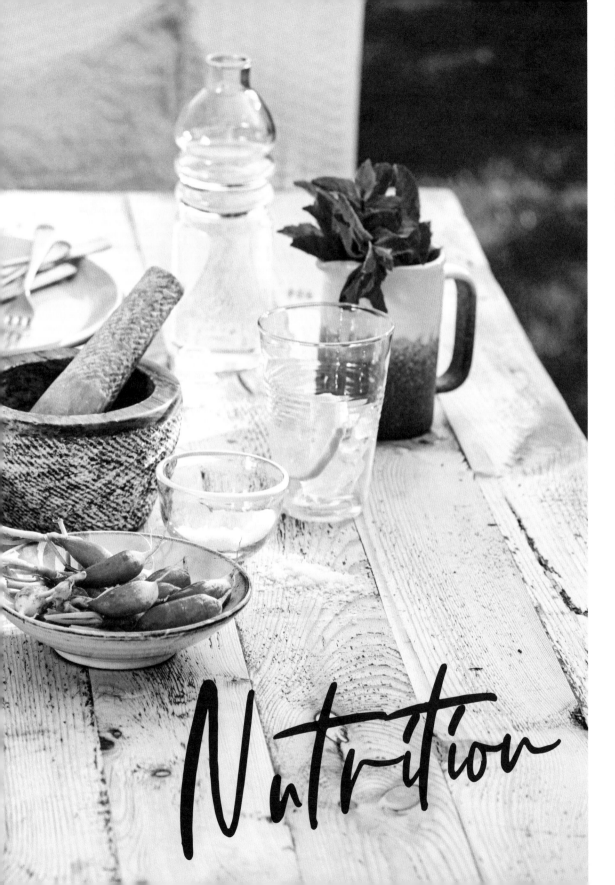

Nutrition

Eat Less, work out more?

When we are talking about our attitude to fitness and food, I think there can often be conflict for people.

In my case I suppose my attitude could best be summed up as all or nothing. On the one hand I can be very disciplined and, when my head wants to focus and make a conscious effort to do something, it definitely will. But when I overindulge, I recognise it can be a slippery slope and one I need to control. I believe food has as much emphasis on how we look and feel as exercise does, and though exercise is a huge part, you can definitely see bigger gains and quicker results if you concentrate on your food.

The right diet helps every part of us feel its best – good skin, healthy hair, lower body fat, more energy, increased strength and focus – it has a 360° effect that goes far beyond just seeing a decreasing number on the scales.

Of course, being a former athlete and into my fitness means that I find it much easier to physically 'beast' my body than to restrict my food intake. But, even with my high fitness levels and stamina, I know that making healthier food choices and creating balance in my daily food intake makes all the difference. What I want you to take from this food section is the ability to really manage your food intake in a way that enhances every part of your life. No one wants to live a life of denial, it's all about finding that magical happy spot called moderation.

Nutrients

Antioxidants are crucial for post-exercise recovery to neutralise free radicals and tissue damage, thus reducing inflammation. Some vital functions of common antioxidants, such as vitamins A, C, D and E as well as zinc are listed below. B vitamins – B1, B2, B3, B5, B6, B9, B12 – and biotin are all essential for the metabolism of carbohydrates and fats for energy. Many also help regulate blood sugar.

VITAMIN A is essential for epithelial tissue repair and regeneration, enhances phagocytes and antibody production (boosting the immune system) and maintains myelin sheath (neurones) and mucous membrane integrity. Good food sources: yellow, red and green vegetables, carrots, sweet potatoes and eggs.

NIACIN (B3) helps maintain healthy skin and nerves. It also has cholesterol-lowering effects at higher doses. Find it in chicken, salmon, prawns, sweet potatoes, sunflower seeds, carrots and tomatoes.

FOLATE (B9) works with vitamin B12 to help form red blood cells. It is needed for the production of DNA, which controls tissue growth and cell function. Find it in lentils, asparagus, spinach, broccoli, avocado, quinoa, strawberries, raspberries and pineapple.

VITAMIN B6 is also called pyridoxine. It helps form red blood cells and maintain brain function. Good food sources: tuna, turkey, chicken, salmon, sweet potatoes, asparagus, avocado, leeks, tomatoes, sunflower seeds, spinach and bananas.

VITAMIN B12, like the other B vitamins, is important for metabolism. It also helps form red blood cells and maintain the central nervous system. Find it in meat, milk, yogurt, cheese, eggs, sardines, salmon, tuna, scallops and prawns.

VITAMIN C Required for connective tissue replacement, red blood cells and adrenaline formation and neutralises free radicals, rejuvenates vitamin E and enhances iron absorption. Good food sources – orange, grapefruit, kiwi, strawberries, tomatoes, red peppers, broccoli, potatoes and spinach.

VITAMIN D Essential for immunity and endocrine regulation. Good food sources include fatty fish, beef, egg yolks and cheese.

VITAMIN E Protects cell membranes, enhances T-helper cell synthesis (helping the immune system), neutralises free radicals, improves blood flow, reduces inflammation. Good food sources: organic pure vegetable oils, (avocado, wheat germ), nuts, seeds and green leafy veg.

ZINC Essential for DNA and RNA synthesis, every aspect of immunity, testosterone production, insulin and growth hormones synthesis. It also reduces lactic acid levels, aids wound healing and influences essential hormone release. Good food sources: poultry, red meat, especially venison, chickpeas, cashew nuts and almonds.

What is a healthy balanced diet?

A good diet is important for our health and helps us feel our best – but what is a good diet? No single food contains all the essential nutrients the body needs to stay healthy and work properly, apart from breast milk as a food for babies! For this reason, our diets should contain a variety of different foods to help us get the wide range of nutrients that our bodies need. This is illustrated by the UK's healthy eating model – the Eatwell Guide.

›› BALANCE

Balance is defined as bringing elements into harmony. If you think of elements as 'food' and harmony as the 'healthy body' then that's when we will achieve a truly balanced body. I think this should be the ultimate goal when it comes to both nutrition and exercise.

What balance is not about is denial and that's why restricting what we eat isn't helpful – we need fuel to live and perform.

Just like your car that requires petrol, oil and electric to run, our body needs carbohydrates, proteins and fats to function properly, so cutting out whole food groups will never help us achieve the best from our bodies.

But, that said, depending on the kind of training you do and your fitness goals, the energy and the recovery time you need will probably determine which food groups you draw the most calories from.

›› ENERGY

We all need energy to grow, stay alive, keep warm and be active and that energy is provided by the carbohydrate, protein and fat in the foods and drinks we consume. It is also provided by alcohol. Different food and drinks provide different amounts of energy. You can find this information on food labels when they are present.

Energy is measured in units of kilocalories (kcal) or kilojoules (kJ) One kilocalorie (1 kcal) is equal to 4.18 kilojoules (4.18 kJ).

FAT contains 9 KCAL (37 KJ) PER GRAM

ALCOHOL contains 7 KCAL (29 KJ) PER GRAM

PROTEIN contains 4 KCAL (17 KJ) PER GRAM

CARBOHYDRATE contains 3.75 KCAL (16 KJ) PER GRAM (for the purposes of food labelling this is rounded up to 4 kcal per gram)

- ### ENERGY REQUIREMENTS
  Carbohydrate is the most important source of energy for the body because it is the main fuel for both your muscles and brain. Sources of carbohydrate include starchy foods, e.g. bread, rice, potatoes, pasta, pulses and breakfast cereals. Choose higher fibre and wholegrain versions of these where possible.

  Different people need different amounts of energy. The amount needed to maintain a healthy weight depends on your basal metabolic rate (BMR), which is the minimum amount of energy your body uses to maintain the basic bodily functions like breathing and your heart beat. BMR varies from person to person depending on your age, body size, gender` and genes. But we also use energy to digest food and for physical activity.

- ### ENERGY BALANCE
  Your weight depends on the balance between how much energy you consume from food and drinks, and the total amount of energy that is used by your body. When you eat or drink more energy than you use, you put on weight; if you consume less energy from your diet than you use, you lose weight; but if you eat and drink the same amount of energy as you use up, you are in energy balance and your weight remains the same. It is important for your health to maintain a healthy weight.

ENERGY IN = calories taken in from food and drink.

ENERGY OUT = calories used by the body for physical activity and other bodily processes such as heart rate and breathing.

›› CARBOHYDRATES

There are two types of carbohydrates: simple, high-glycaemic index carbohydrates, and complex, low-glycaemic index carbohydrates. But which one is best pre-workout?

This ultimately depends on your goal and the time of your pre-workout meal. Simple carbohydrates are great for 30 minutes to an hour before a workout, as they provide the body with fast-acting glucose as fuel. However, complex carbohydrates also play a role within energy metabolism. By consuming low GI carbohydrates around 2–3 hours before a workout, you can give your body a slow-releasing source of energy. This means you'll be able to work out for longer and be less likely to have a dip in your blood sugar levels in the middle of your workout.

›› PROTEINS

Protein is especially important to consume after a workout as, during exercise, you are effectively breaking your muscles down. That is why it's a common sight to see people at the gym eating protein bars or drinking whey shakes when they have finished their routine – it helps to increase the impact of their exercise. It's also important to mix this protein with carbohydrates as your body finds it easier to absorb the protein and turn it into more muscle mass when carbohydrate is present.

Pre-workout meals containing protein can also give your body the amino acids (branched-chain amino acids in particular) that it needs to prevent muscle breakdown, while aiding muscle recovery and growth. However, athletes and people who regularly lift weights may find that they may need to add protein powders to their diet to help maximise muscle gain and fat loss. Protein powders are concentrated sources of animal or plant

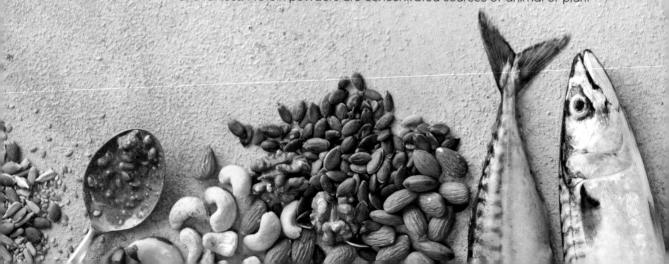

protein, such as dairy, eggs, rice or peas. It's important to note that not everyone will benefit from taking supplements. If your diet is already rich in high-quality protein, it's likely you won't see much difference simply by adding protein powder. There are about seven different types of protein powder and I have used whey, egg, pea and brown rice.

Whey protein powder is quickly digested, providing a rapid rise in amino acids that may help increase muscle mass and strength. Eggs are a well-known source of high-quality protein and egg white protein is also easily digested and absorbed. Pea protein powder is especially popular among vegetarians and vegans. It's made from yellow split peas, which contain high amounts of all the essential amino acids except for methionine. Brown rice protein powder contains all of the essential amino acids but is too low in lysine to be considered a complete protein.

›› FATS

During high-intensity exercise, where carbohydrate is the main fuel source, fat is needed to help access the stored carbohydrate (glycogen). The body needs to break down fat and transport it to the working muscles before it can be used as energy. Fats take longer to break down into energy your body can use, while carbohydrates are easily broken down into energy. This is why your body uses fat at rest – when it has time to get the energy – and carbohydrate during intense exercise – when you need a lot of energy quickly. Replacing the refined carbohydrates in your everyday diet with 'good' fats will improve your body's ability to burn fat for energy rather than carbohydrate even when exercising.

It seems that fat could be the way forward for sustained energy throughout the day. What's more, foods that contain good fats tend to come packaged with lots of other nutrients we need, unlike refined carbohydrates. Try avocado, walnuts, oily fish, raw virgin coconut oil, olive oil or flaxseeds.

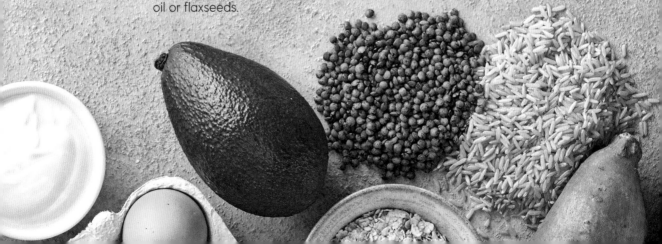

5 WAYS TO IMPROVE THE WAY YOU EAT

1. ENJOY BREAKFAST

Many people believe that skipping breakfast will help cut calories from their daily intake and, therefore, shed pounds. But it also has a huge impact on your performance throughout the day, as people who miss breakfast tend to feel fatigued early on and have low concentration levels, affecting their efficiency.

2. HEALTHY SNACKING

Healthy snacking plays a pivotal role in overall health and wellbeing. By snacking on good nutritious foods, our bodies and minds feel the benefits. Healthy snacking helps curb cravings, helps with weight management, regulates mood, boosts brain power and gives you the energy that you need to power through your day. Healthy snacks include: dates, blueberries, figs, cucumber sticks, apples, nuts and many more.

3. MINDFUL EATING

I admit I have a sweet tooth but I am mindful of that. In order to become fit and healthy, you need to be eating real foods. Portion control is key and it's imperative that you are drinking plenty of water. Fizzy drinks and endless booze will harm you morethan they will help you in the long run. Opt for fresh food, not fast food. Add fruits, vegetables, and healthy snacks and begin to phase out processed food and calorific 'treats'.

4. DRINK MORE WATER

When your body is hydrated, you are giving it the chance to work at its optimum level. By drinking a minimum of 2 litres of water per day (3 litres if working out), you will benefit from: increased energy levels and less fatigue, a boosted immune system, healthier skin, improved mood and much more.

5. MONITOR HOW MUCH PROCESSED FOODS YOU EAT

Lots of people enjoy junk food now and again, mainly because it is cheap, but in order to lead a healthy life, it is vital that you watch how much processed food you're eating. Processed foods are chemically altered to give them their taste and, when consumed frequently, they can cause a variety of issues. These include: mood swings, sleep loss, weight gain and addiction to processed foods. So be mindful of how much you are eating.

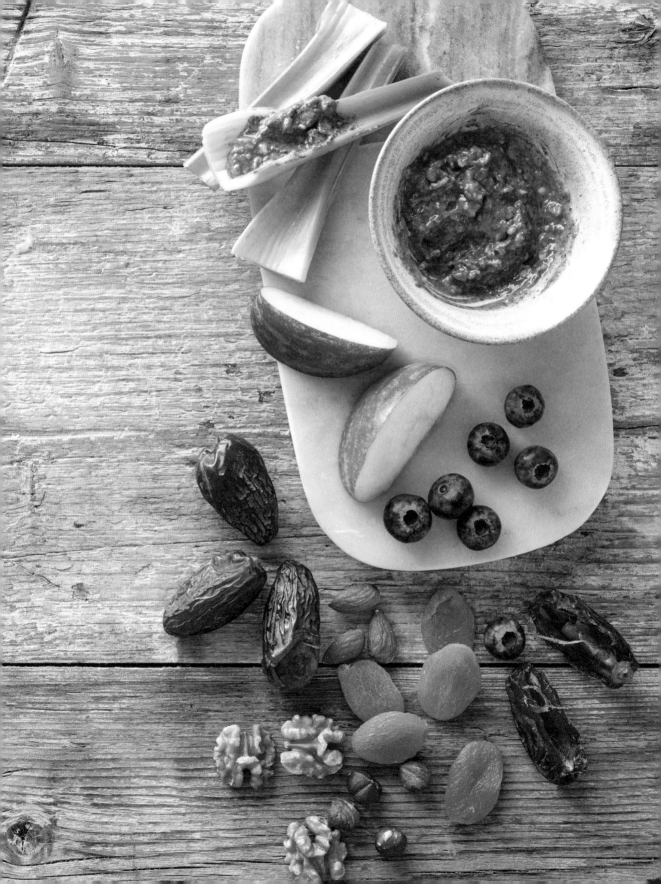

Food for performance

Eating for training results shouldn't just take place after the gym or right before a big sporting event. If you want to see proper results and continuous progress then it is something you should be conscious of when consuming every meal and every snack. You have to be honest with yourself because you really do only get out what you put in. Your strategy should obviously involve more whole and natural foods than the manufactured kind, such as protein bars and drinks, although I admit I do eat and drink them as a quick fix and they do play their part in helping achieve instant recovery.

HERE ARE EIGHT OF MY FAVOURITE FOODS WHEN I AM IN THE 'TRAINING ZONE' AND WANT TO BETTER MY PERFORMANCE:

1 QUINOA
Although it's really a sprouted seed, quinoa is usually considered a whole grain — and a great one at that. It's got nearly twice as much protein (8 grams per cup) as other grains, and it's one of the few plant foods to contain all nine essential amino acids our bodies need to build lean muscle and recover from tough workouts. Quinoa's also a great source of fibre and carbohydrates.

2 BERRIES
Antioxidants such as vitamins A, C, and E help protect against oxidative stress and free radicals that form in the body during strenuous physical activity — and berries are one of the best sources of antioxidants out there. Choose berries with the darkest colour like blackberries, blueberries or raspberries.

3 FISH
Oily fish, like salmon, mackerel and trout, are good sources of lean protein and omega-3 fatty acids, which help reduce inflammation that can hamper athletic performance.

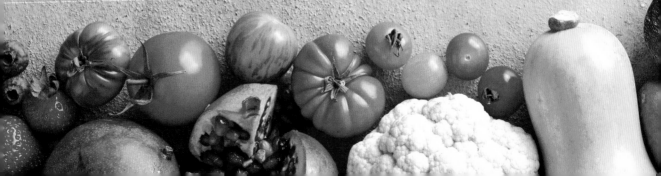

4 BEANS AND LEGUMES

For vegetarian athletes (or those who just want to go meatless once in a while), plant-based sources of protein are a must. These include soybeans, tofu, lentils, peas, and all beans – like black, pinto, kidney, etc. Unlike animal protein, beans have no saturated fat and are also a good source of fibre, which can help keep you feeling fuller, longer.

5 GREEN VEGETABLES

All vegetables are good vegetables when it comes to providing the vitamins and minerals your body needs for good performance. However, dark and leafy greens like broccoli, cauliflower, Brussels sprouts and kale have higher amounts of antioxidants, fibre, and other important nutrients.

6 NUTS AND NUT BUTTERS

As they are a natural combination of protein and healthy fats, nuts are great for people who work out a lot. They're easy to digest and can help balance your blood sugar when paired with carbs. I love peanut or almond butter on toast, because the protein and fat can help slow the release of the carbs from the toast, keeping you fuller for longer.

7 CHOCOLATE MILK

Some people mistakenly think you need a lot of protein after a workout. However, what works best are simple carbs mixed with a little bit of protein. So a glass of low-fat chocolate milk can get the same benefits as a protein overload. Also, the caffeine in the chocolate dilates and relaxes blood vessels, helping oxygen-rich blood reach your muscles quicker.

8 BANANAS

Bananas contain sugar and natural electrolytes. They are not as convenient as bars or gels, but they are a good option if you want a natural, less-processed alternative. One banana contains just over 400mg potassium, which your body needs to regulate fluids and prevent muscle cramps. Because you sweat out potassium during physical activity, it's important to replenish as soon as possible afterwards.

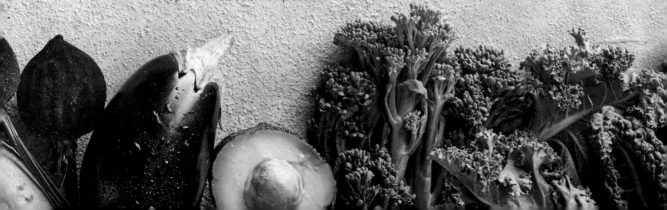

Eating and running

Eating right before and after your run can make a massive difference to your experience and/or end result. Here are some of the tips and principles that I follow:

›› SHOULD I BE EATING THE SAME FOR ALL MY RUNS?

Your body requires different fuel depending on the type of training.

During harder training sessions and races, your body uses carbohydrates (stored in the muscles as glycogen) as its main fuel (energy) source. You're only able to store a relatively small amount of carbohydrate, which is why keeping it topped up is so important.

During low-intensity exercise, such as jogging or walking, the body burns fat as its main energy source. Therefore, fuelling with carbohydrates isn't as crucial and a high-protein meal or snack before your run is good. The important thing is to plan which sessions you need to be 'fuelled' with carbs for versus other energy sources.

›› HOW LONG AFTER EATING A MEAL SHOULD I WAIT BEFORE GOING FOR A RUN?

Everyone has different levels of comfort regarding eating around training, so it's important to trial what works best for you. In general, wait 2–3 hours before running after eating a large meal. After a smaller snack, 30–90 minutes should be sufficient, depending on how much you have eaten.

For energy-boosting fuel before a harder run, have smaller carbohydrate snacks that have a reasonably high glycaemic index score (GI). A food's GI measure is relative to how quickly it's digested and broken down into glucose, so high-GI foods are absorbed faster and less strain is placed on the gut. For low-intensity training sessions that last under an hour, the occasional fasted session is fine and can help the muscles to become more efficient for endurance training.

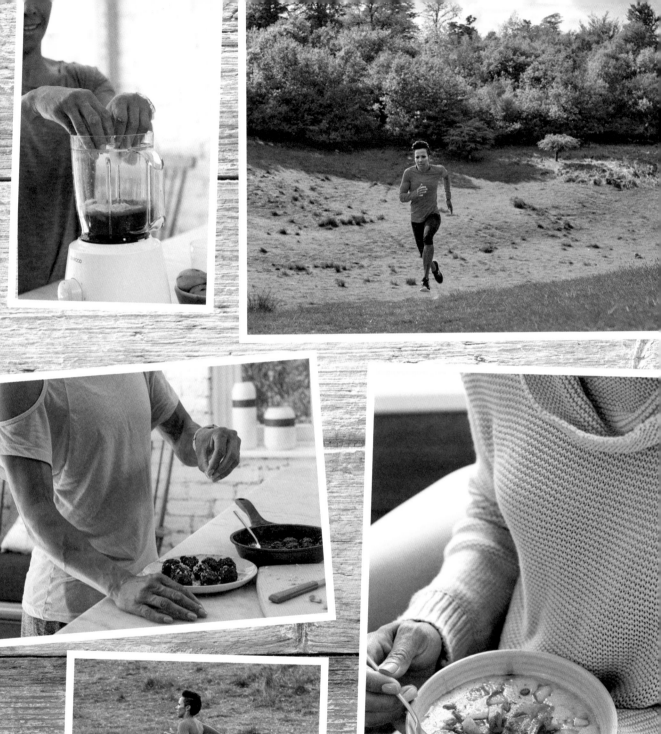

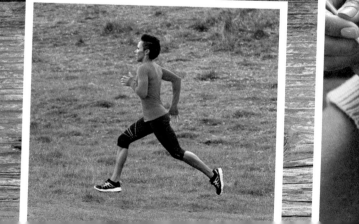

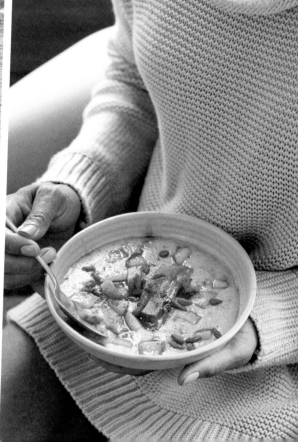

>> SHOULD I EAT BEFORE AN EARLY MORNING RUN AND IF SO, WHAT?

You should always plan to eat before a harder training session, as the body will require fuel from carbohydrates. For lighter, low-intensity training, a protein-based breakfast or even a fasted training session are fine.

THERE ARE THREE MORNING SITUATIONS TO PLAN FOR:

1. the early riser

If you wake up 2 hours before your run, good options include oats (page 175), quinoa or cinnamon porridge, blueberry pancakes, wholegrain toast topped with eggs, granola, bagels or breakfast muffins (page 168) and freshly made smoothies (pages 182–187).

2. straight out of bed

If like me, you prefer to get straight on the road, try a small snack with quick-releasing energy, such energy balls (pages 192–194), fruit or a small flapjack (page 190).

If you struggle to eat first thing, try increasing the carbohydrate portion of your evening meal the night before, as this will be stored in the muscles ready for your morning run.

3. 'training low'

This is a new strategy used by professional athletes to help the muscles adapt to endurance training. For a low-intensity endurance session, you may plan to reduce the carbs in your breakfast as this can encourage the body to burn fat for fuel.

>> WHAT SHOULD I DEFINITELY AVOID EATING BEFORE A RUN?

To provide sufficient fuel, foods should be mostly high in carbohydrate, but you should also eat foods that you're used to and that don't feel too 'heavy' in your stomach when you begin exercising. In the 2–3 hours before a run, try to avoid the following as these are well-known causes of gastrointestinal distresses such as diarrhoea and bowel upsets.

WHAT TO AVOID
- Foods very high in fibre
- Excessively fatty foods
- Unusually spicy foods
- Drinking too much caffeine
- Alcohol

›› ON THE MORNING OF A BIG RACE, WHEN SHOULD I EAT AND WHAT SHOULD I OPT FOR?

What you eat on the morning of your event should be the same as your normal fuelling strategy that you have for training. Eat a meal 2–3 hours before the start of the race, and include a range of foods depending on your taste.

GOOD BREAKFAST OPTIONS INCLUDE:
- Pancakes and mixed toppings, such as fruits and nuts
- Porridge oats with milk or soy milk
- Granola with milk or soy milk
- Multigrain toast topped with eggs
- Fruit salad and low-fat Greek yogurt
- Bagels or breakfast muffins with low-fat cottage cheese or peanut butter
- Fruit juice or a fruit smoothie (pages 182–187)

As a general rule, low-GI foods are best eaten as part of your main meals while training (alongside moderate amounts of protein and fat), as their energy is released more slowly and will provide you with sustained energy. For a low-GI breakfast see page 168, low-GI lunch see page 200 and low-GI dinner see page 215.

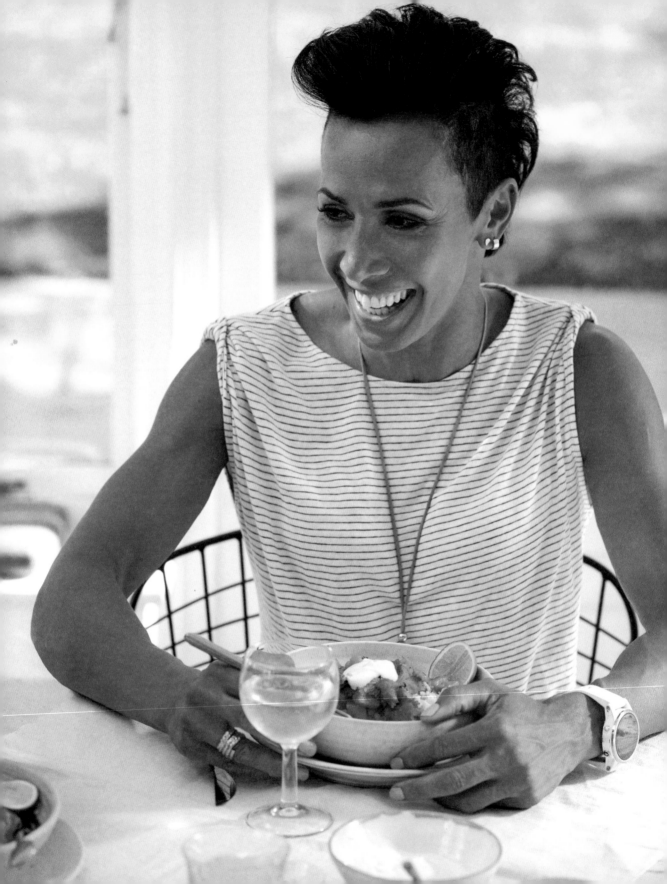

my
recipes

Winner's breakfast egg muffins

serves 6

450g butternut squash, peeled and cut into 3cm chunks
2 tablespoons olive oil
60g spinach
4 spring onions, finely sliced
12 large eggs
1 teaspoon ground turmeric
½ teaspoon freshly ground black pepper
chilli flakes or pul biber (*optional*)

Turmeric has several health benefits including anti-inflammatory, antioxidant and anti-cancer properties. It is a good source of manganese and contains iron, vitamin B6, fibre, copper and potassium. Curcumin is the principle active ingredient in turmeric and gives it its vibrant colour. Add black pepper to any dish prepared with turmeric for better absorption as it contains piperine, a natural substance that enhances the absorption of curcumin by up to 2000%.

Preheat the oven to 180°C/gas mark 4.

Spread out the butternut squash on a roasting tray, drizzle with the oil and season. Roast for 20–30 minutes.

Remove from the oven and mix together with the spinach and spring onions in a large bowl. Divide the vegetables between the holes of a 12-hole muffin tray.

Whisk the eggs, turmeric, pepper and chilli flakes together in a bowl. Pour over the vegetables in the muffin tray.

Reduce the oven temperature to 150°C/gas mark 2 and bake the muffins for 30 minutes until they are puffed and golden.

These can be also be served with lean grilled bacon, if you wish. They will keep for a couple of days in the fridge.

NUTRITION

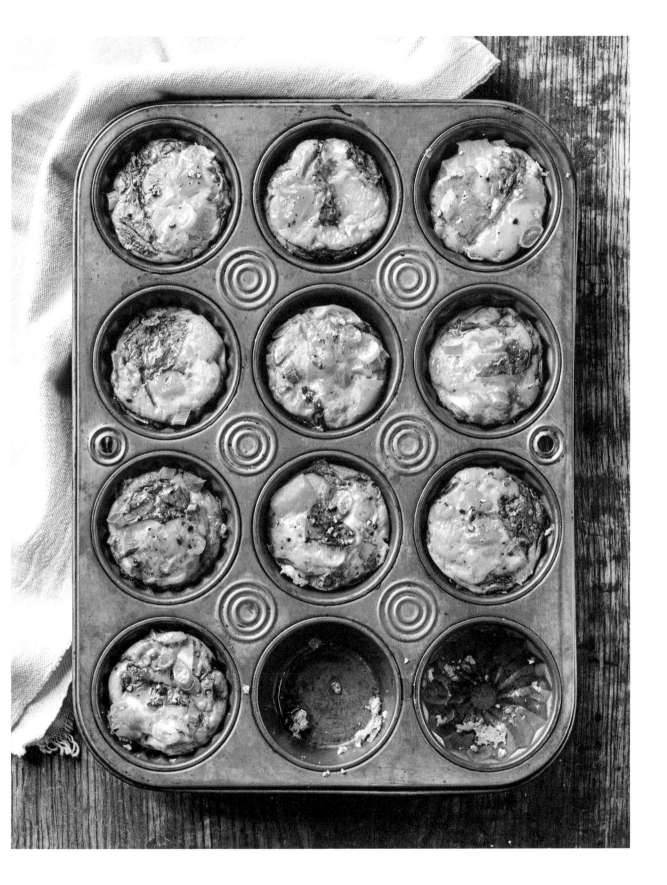

Cacao chia breakfast treat

serves 4

8 tablespoons chia seeds
400ml coconut milk
200ml almond milk
1 tablespoon lemon juice
150g quark, plain yogurt or
  Skyr
50g dark chocolate (approx.
  80% cocoa solids)
150g granola
2 tablespoons cacao powder
1 teaspoon honey or maple
  syrup
sprigs of mint, to garnish

Raw cacoa helps reduce the oxidative stress of strenuous activities because of the high magnesium, B vitamin and antioxidant content, so these cacao chia pots make a great breakfast after a workout.

Mix the chia seeds, coconut milk and almond milk together and refrigerate for a minimum of 3 hours or overnight if possible.

Mix the lemon juice into the quark or yogurt and put it in the fridge to chill.

Melt the chocolate in a heatproof bowl over a saucepan of barely simmering water. Add half the granola, stir to coat in the chocolate and chill.

Remove the chia mixture from the fridge and stir in the cacao powder and honey or maple syrup.

Line four small glasses or pots with honey and layer in the cacao-chia mix, the remaining granola and lemon quark and top with the chocolate granola. Garnish with a sprig of mint on top of each serving.

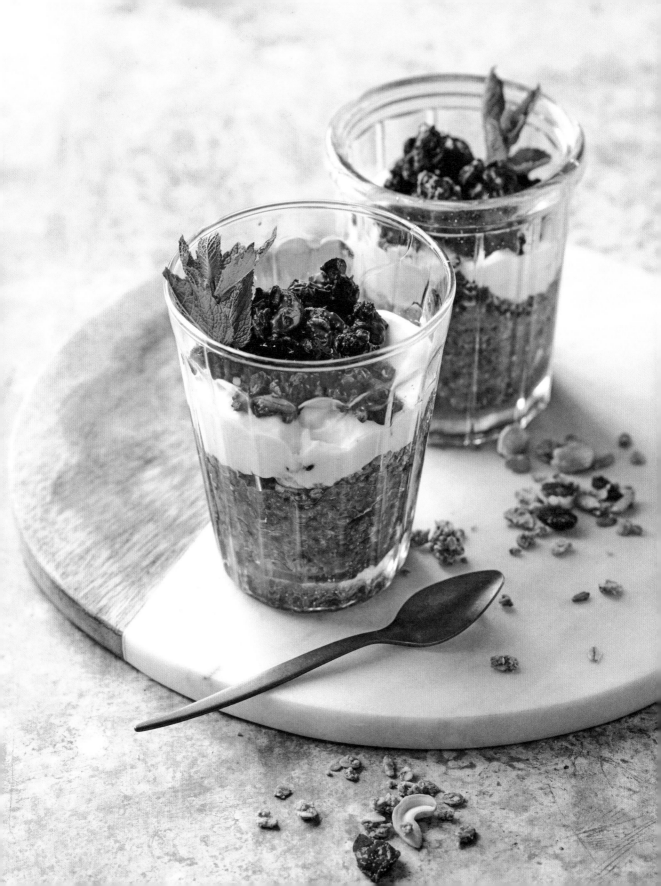

Warm breakfast salad bowl

serves 2

FOR THE SALAD

400g butternut squash (approx. 1 large butternut), peeled and cut into bite-size chunks

2 tablespoons olive oil, plus extra for crispy kale

200g aubergine (approx. 1 large aubergine), cut into bite-size chunks

1 large red pepper, deseeded and sliced

100g mushrooms (4–5 breakfast mushrooms), sliced

30g kale

sea salt and freshly ground black pepper

FOR THE DRESSING

1 tablespoon lemon juice

½ teaspoon maple syrup

3 tablespoons coconut oil

chilli flakes or pul biber

TO SERVE

crispy kale and/or poached egg

Eggs are a great source of inexpensive, high-quality protein. The whites are packed with selenium, vitamin D, B6, B12 and minerals such as zinc and iron while the yolks contain vitamins A, D, E and K. So top these colourful vegetables with a poached egg and some nutrient-rich kale for a healthy and filling breakfast bowl.

Preheat the oven to 180°C/gas mark 4.

Put the butternut squash into a roasting dish and drizzle with half the oil then season with salt and pepper. Bake for 10 minutes then add the aubergine and red pepper, drizzle with the remaining oil and return to the oven for a further 5 minutes. Remove from the oven and add the mushrooms, then roast for a further 15 minutes or until all the vegetables are softened and beginning to caramelise around the edges. If serving with crispy kale, spread the kale onto a baking tray, drizzle with oil and bake for 15–20 minutes.

Meanwhile, poach the egg. Crack the egg into a ramekin. Heat a pan of boiling water, about 6-8 cm deep. Add a glug of vinegar and whisk frantically to create a swirl, then lower egg in. Use a large slotted spoon to gather in the stray bits of white towards the egg to make it as neat as possible. They will all vary in shape. If the white separates too much, the egg is not fresh enough.

To make the dressing, mix all the ingredients together in a small bowl.

Serve with poached egg and/or crispy kale. Drizzle over the dressing or serve on the side.

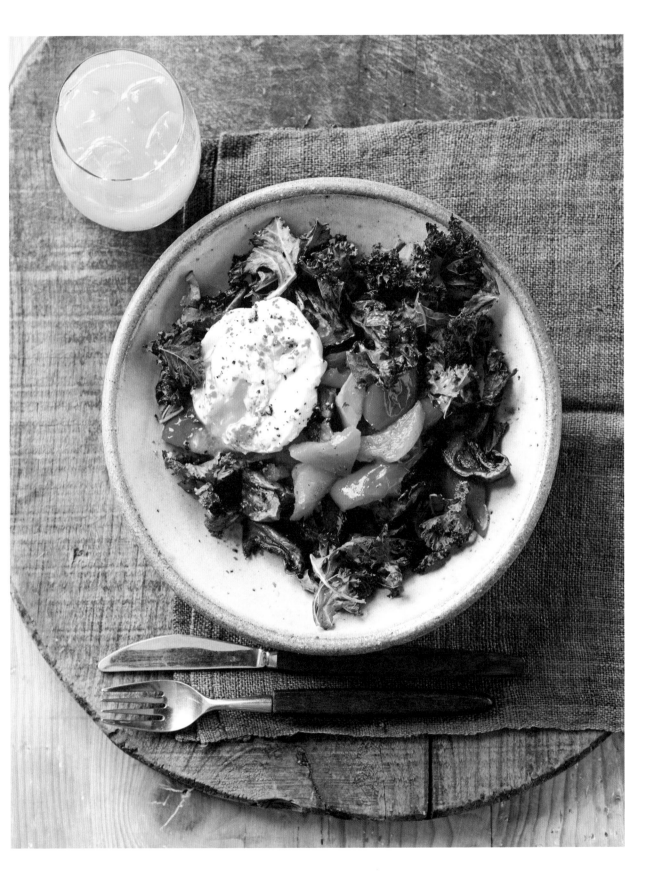

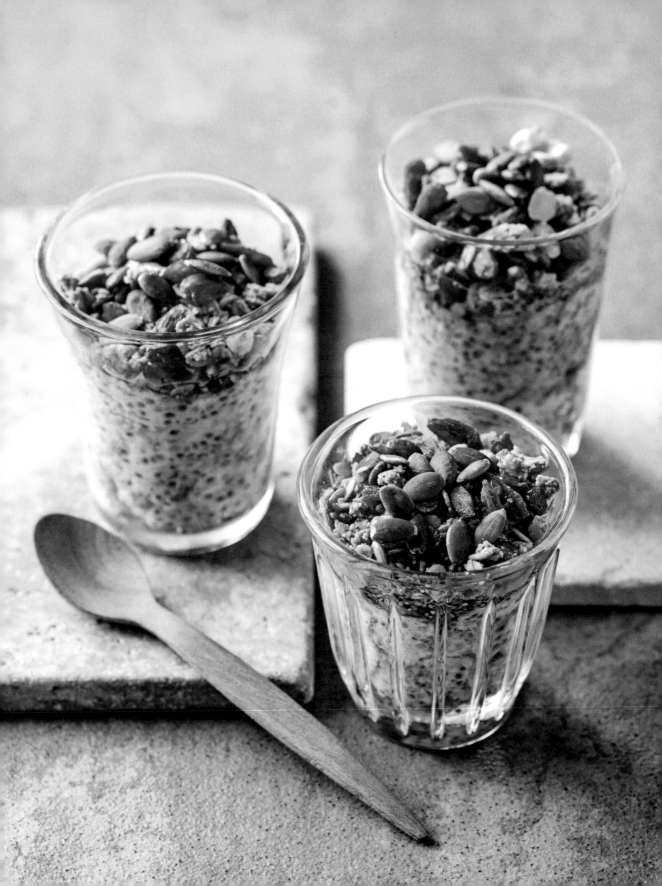

Vanilla & almond overnight oats

serves 4

60g oats

4 tablespoons chia seeds

200ml almond milk, plus
3–4 tablespoons

1 teaspoon vanilla extract

runny honey

4 tablespoons granola

2 tablespoons goji berries

2 tablespoons pumpkin seeds

1 teaspoon almond butter
(*optional*)

Chia seeds were originally grown in Mexico. Aztec and Mayan warriors ate them for fuel during battle or when running long distances. They are energy-boosting, nutrient-dense and an excellent source of essential fatty acids. They are a good source of vitamins A, B1 and B3, E and D, iron, iodine, magnesium and manganese.

Soak the oats and chia seeds in the almond milk and vanilla extract and refrigerate for 4 hours or overnight if possible.

Remove the oat and chia mixture from the fridge and add 3–4 tablespoons of almond milk to loosen the mix slightly.

Drizzle a little honey inside four glasses. Divide the oat and chia seed mixture evenly between each glass, top with the granola, goji berries and pumpkin seeds and drizzle with extra honey, if you wish. You can also top with a little almond butter for an extra nutty flavour, if you like.

Açaí berry bowl

serves 2

100g pouch açaí, frozen
1 peeled and frozen banana
juice of ½ orange
2 tablespoons organic
    natural or Greek yogurt
1 tablespoon mixed seeds,
    such as pumpkin, sunflower
    or sesame
a handful of mixed berries,
    such as blueberries,
    raspberries or strawberries
drizzle of honey (*optional*)

Açaí, the Brazilian superfood, is particularly high in antioxidants, which protect your body from inflammation and free radical cellular damage. They also aid muscular repair so are good for those exercising. The berries are a good source of calcium and fibre too. You can buy them frozen from health stores or online for your convenience. Add a little of your favourite protein powder if you'd like to boost the protein content of this breakfast bowl. This also makes a perfect pre- or post-workout smoothie if you are short of time.

Put the açaí, banana and orange juice into a food processor or high-speed blender and blend until smooth.

Spoon into two bowls and top with the yogurt, seeds and berries and drizzle with honey, if you wish. Alternatively blend all the ingredients together in a high-speed blender and enjoy as a smoothie on the go.

Pinhead oatmeal with figs, nuts & honey

serves 2

100g pinhead porridge oats
   or rolled porridge oats
2 tablespoons goji berries
   (*optional*)
2 tablespoons chopped
   walnuts
2 tablespoons pumpkin seeds
400ml almond milk
   (or 200ml milk and 200ml
   water)
salt
2 tablespoons flaxseed,
   freshly ground
4 fresh juicy figs, chopped
   (dried if unavailable)
1 banana, peeled and sliced
raw honey, to drizzle

Pinhead oats have a lovely nutty texture, but you can use regular oatmeal if you prefer, it will just need a little less cooking time. Nuts, seeds and oats are a perfect energy-sustaining breakfast combo of protein and slow-releasing carbohydrate. Soaking the nuts and seeds makes them easier to digest.

Flaxseeds add essential omega 3 fats. Goji berries and figs are packed with vitamins, minerals and antioxidants. Bananas are rich in potassium, magnesium and fibre, but more importantly their carb content is the perfect energy boost for a pre-workout breakfast.

Soak the oats, goji berries if using, walnuts and pumpkin seeds in the milk in the fridge overnight.

In the morning, pour the mixture into a saucepan, add 200ml water and a pinch of salt and bring to the boil. Simmer gently for 3–4 minutes until creamy in texture. Add a splash more almond milk or water to loosen the mixture if necessary.

Divide between two bowls and top with the ground flaxseed, fruit and honey.

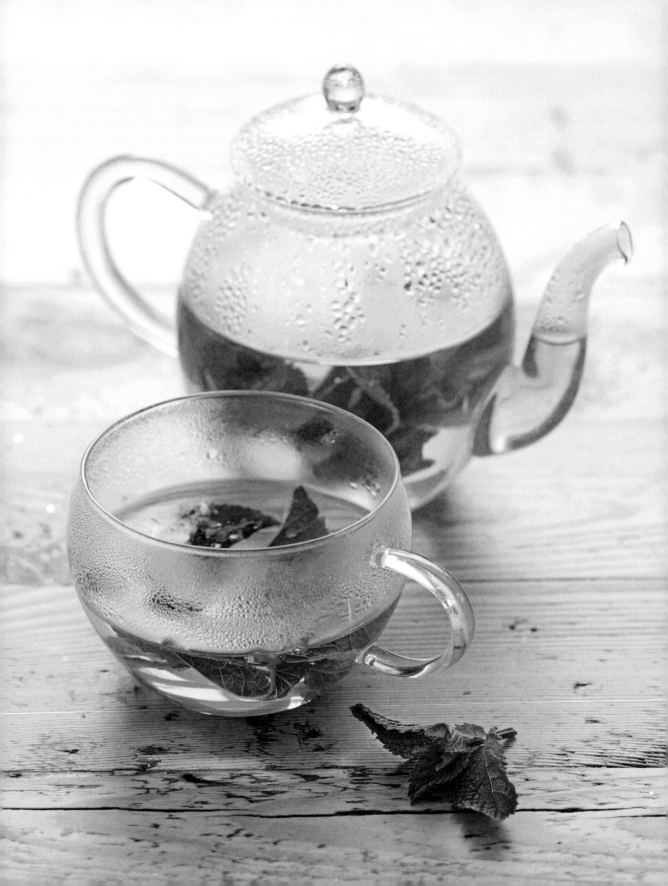

Fresh mint & lemon infusion

serves 1

approx. 5 mint leaves
1 slice of lemon

Fresh mint helps with digestion and can soothe an upset stomach so a refreshing mint tea is the perfect drink to enjoy after a meal.

Put the mint leaves and lemon slice into a mug and pour over boiling water.

Turmeric, cayenne & black pepper twist

serves 2

2 tablespoons cider vinegar
2 tablespoons lemon juice
½ teaspoon ground turmeric
   or grated fresh turmeric
½ teaspoon black pepper
1 teaspoon honey
cayenne pepper

Turmeric is a good source of curcumin, known for its anti-inflammatory effects and is used in the treatment of numerous inflammatory conditions.

Mix the cider vinegar, lemon juice, turmeric, black pepper and honey in 500ml boiling water. Pour into two mugs and add a little cayenne pepper to taste

RUNNING LIFE

Goji & lemon tea

serves 1

1 teaspoon goji berries
1 slice of lemon

Goji berries contain eighteen types of amino acid, the building blocks of protein, including all eight essential amino acids. These body-building proteins also support brain health and function.

Soak the goji berries and lemon in a mug with a little hot water for at least 1 minute. Add 90 per cent boiling water and 10 per cent cold water.

Ginger & lemon infusion

serves 1

2cm piece of fresh ginger, sliced
1 slice of lemon

Ginger aids digestion and can help to relieve stomach aches and nausea. It is also a powerful anti-inflammatory and antioxidant. It boosts the immune system and has anti-cancer properties.

Put the ginger and lemon into a mug and pour over boiling water.

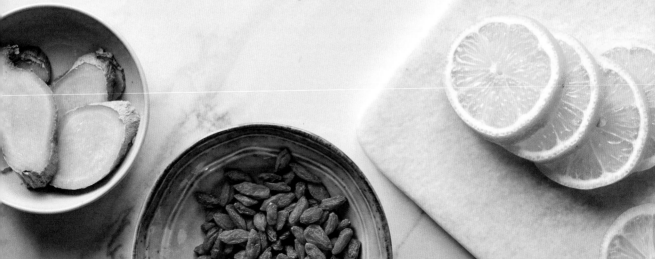

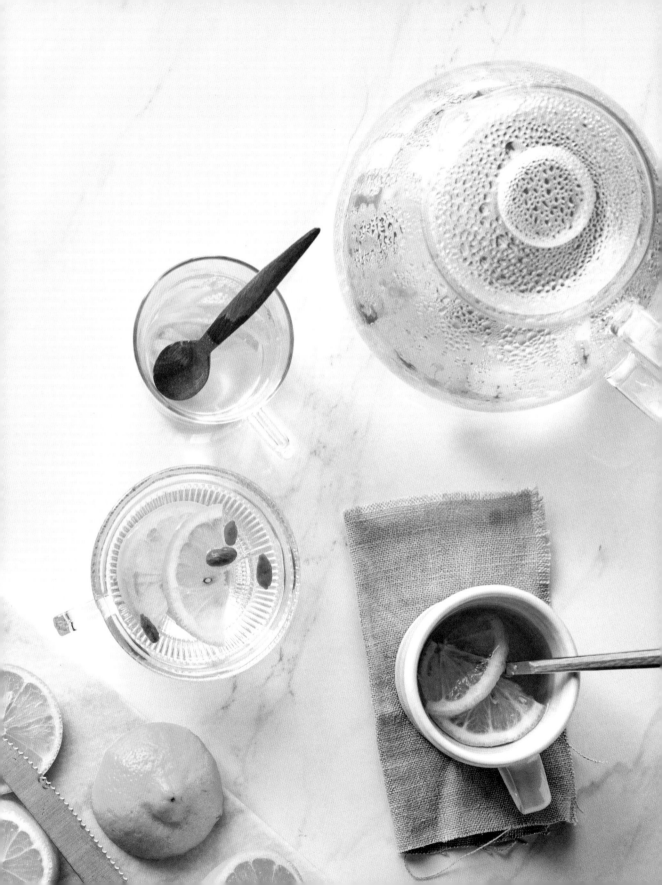

Chocolate dream smoothie

serves 1

1 tablespoon raw cacao
2–3 dates
nut milk of your choice
20g cashew nuts
cacao nibs and bee pollen,
    to serve

This smoothie tastes indulgent but is actually full of nourishing ingredients. Raw cacao (unroasted cocoa) contains one of the highest antioxidant levels of any food as well as magnesium for energy and focus. Dates are nutrient-dense, naturally sweet and packed with fibre to help maintain healthy digestion.

Place all the ingredients in a high-speed blender and blend until smooth. Pour into a glass and top with a sprinkling of cacao nibs and bee pollen.

Breakfast smoothie

serves 1

200ml coconut milk
1 small scoop of granola
1 tablespoon mixed nuts
½ banana, peeled and
    roughly chopped
1 teaspoon maca powder
1 teaspoon honey
1 tablespoon cacao powder,
    plus extra to serve
a handful of ice cubes
chia seeds, to serve

The energy-boosting maca combined with magnesium-and-iron-rich cacao powder in this recipe make this a great smoothie to start your day.

Pour the coconut milk into a high-speed blender and add the granola, nuts, banana, maca powder, honey and cacao powder. Blend everything together before adding the ice and re-blending. Pour into a glass and sprinkle a little chia seeds and cacao powder over the top.

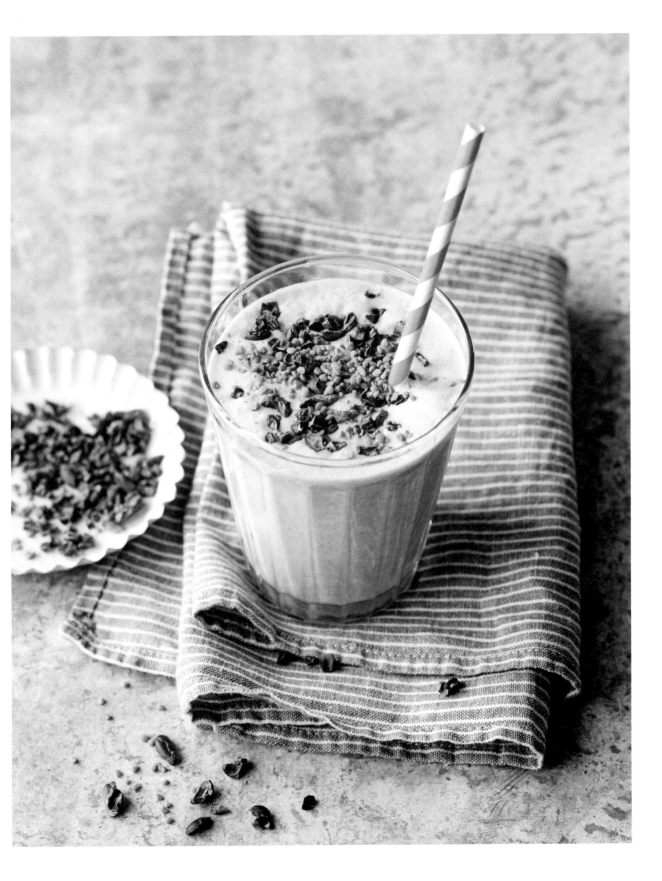

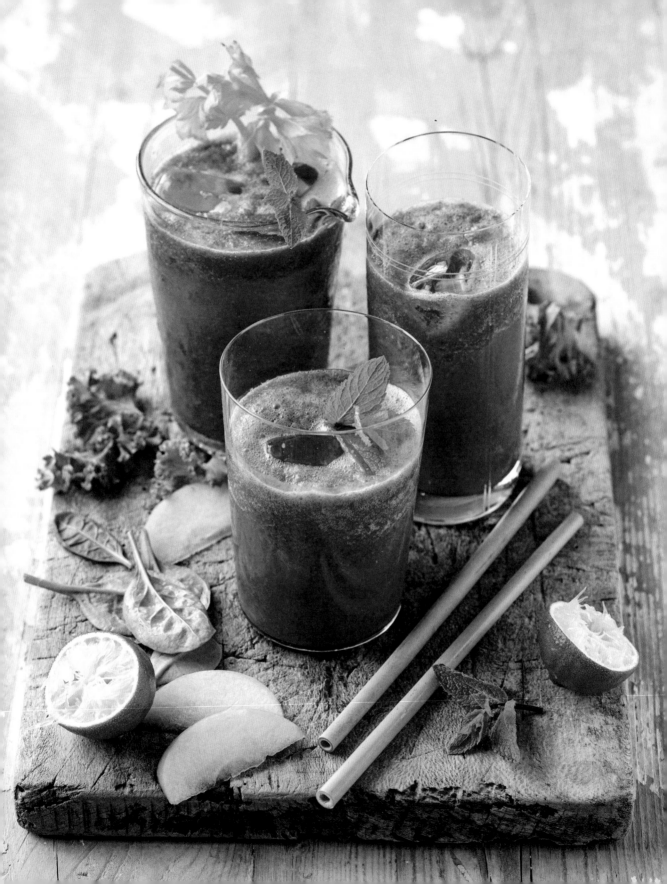

Virtuous green smoothie

serves 1

a handful of spinach
½ stick of celery
2.5cm piece of fresh ginger
juice of ½ lime
1 green apple, cored
½ teaspoon wheatgrass powder
300ml coconut water or water
a handful of ice cubes

This smoothie is cleansing and alkalising. Ginger is useful for treating coughs and colds and also helps settle the stomach. It has anti-inflammatory properties and can boost the metabolism. Wheatgrass is a great detoxifier and a good source of antioxidants.

Place all the ingredients in a high-speed blender and blend until smooth.

Blueberry glow smoothie

serves 1

100g blueberries, plus extra to serve
1 teaspoon baobab
20g oats
¼ avocado, roughly chopped
1 teaspoon hemp seeds
200ml almond milk
a handful of ice cubes
bee pollen, to serve

A great smoothie for the skin and immune system. Baobab is rich in calcium, magnesium and potassium and has ten times more vitamin C than oranges! Avocados contain healthy fats and antioxidants, including vitamin E, which help maintain healthy skin and circulation.

Place all the ingredients in a high-speed blender and blend until smooth. Pour into a glass and top with some extra blueberries and bee pollen.

Beet power smoothie

serves 1

1 small beetroot, scrubbed, topped and tailed and roughly chopped

1 banana, peeled and roughly chopped

1 dessertspoon chia seeds, plus extra to serve

1 teaspoon maca powder

300ml coconut water or water

A perfect pre-workout pick. Beetroot is naturally sweet and contains high levels of beta-carotene and vitamin C to help support immunity, plus iron and folic acid which help prevent fatigue. Potassium-rich maca was used by Incan warriors before battle to help boost energy and stamina. It is also said to support the body when under stress and aid in regulating hormones.

Place all the ingredients in a high-speed blender and blend until smooth. Pour into a glass and top with some extra chia seeds.

Raspberry zinger

serves 1

150ml ginger beer

a handful of raspberries

4 mint leaves

1 teaspoon lemon juice

7.5cm piece of fresh ginger, chopped

a handful of ice cubes

spinach leaf and slice of apple, to garnish (*optional*)

Raspberries are high in vitamin C, which helps the body to absorb iron and maintain healthy tissue, as well as antioxidants. They are also a good source of magnesium and folic acid.

Pour the ginger beer into a high-speed blender. Add the remaining ingredients except the ice and blend until smooth. Add the ice cubes and blend again. Dress with a spinach leaf and slice of apple, if you wish.

Peanut butter & jelly smoothie

serves 1–2

1 tablespoon peanut or almond butter
1 banana, peeled and roughly chopped
1 teaspoon ground cinnamon
200g strawberries
300ml nut milk of your choice
a handful of ice cubes

The perfect energy boost or wholesome treat. Cinnamon can help lower blood sugar levels and contains antioxidants and anti-inflammatory properties and is believed to support a healthy heart. Strawberries are full of antioxidants and dietary fibre to help maintain a healthy body.

Place all the ingredients apart from the ice in a high-speed blender and blend until smooth. Add the ice cubes and blend again.

Super support

serves 1

3 large tomatoes
pinch of sea salt
a handful of flat-leaf parsley
¼ teaspoon cayenne pepper
juice of 1 lemon
1 teaspoon ground turmeric
a handful of ice cubes

This immune-boosting smoothie is perfect if you need a tonic to boost health. Tomatoes contain antioxidants, including beta-carotene, vitamins C and E and zinc, all of which help support a healthy immune system.

Place all the ingredients apart from the ice in a high-speed blender and blend until smooth. Put the ice in a glass and pour over the tomato mixture.

RUNNING LIFE

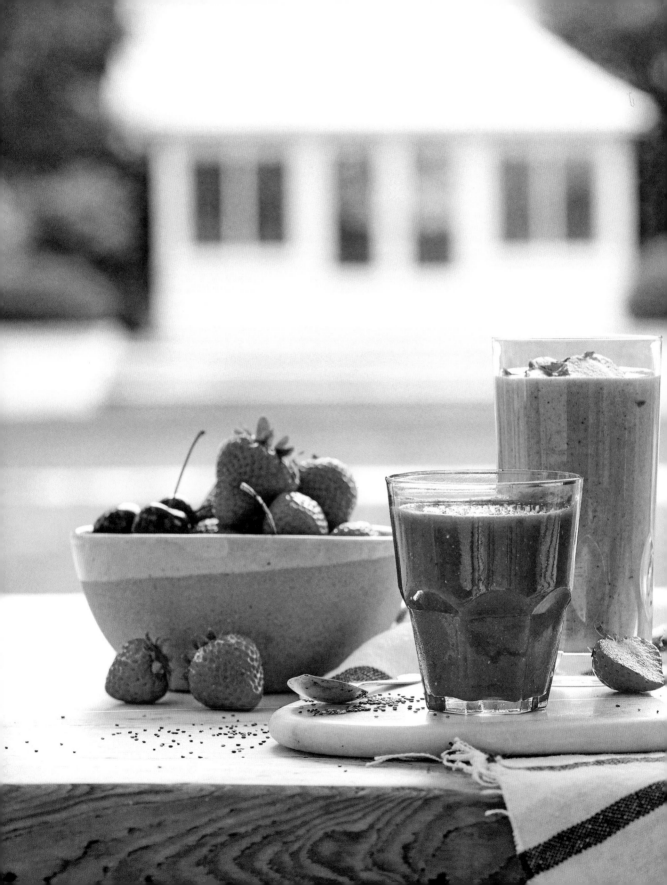

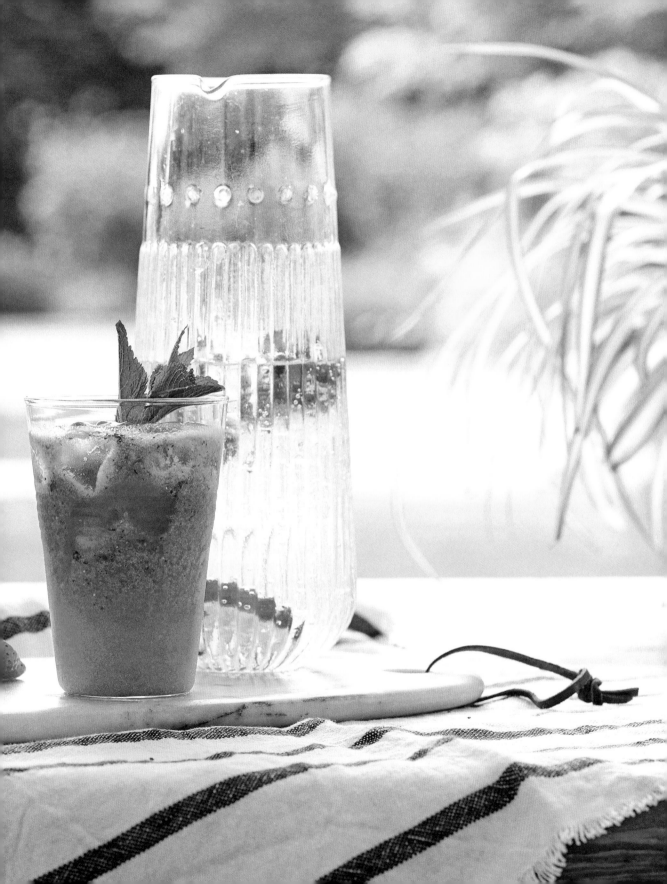

Figgy seeded banana bread

makes 16

250g wholemeal spelt flour

150g coconut sugar or light muscovado

1½ teaspoons baking powder

1 heaped teaspoon Ceylon ground cinnamon

2 very ripe bananas, peeled and mashed

100g dried figs, roughly chopped

100g walnuts, chopped

125ml light olive oil or coconut oil, melted

2 eggs, lightly whisked

50g pumpkin seeds

TO SERVE

sliced banana and peanut butter or cherries and yogurt

This delicious banana bread is packed with protein from the nuts, seeds and wholemeal spelt flour, plus glucose for readily available energy. Small squares of this are a great pre-workout snack, particularly if you need something on the go.

Preheat the oven to 170°C/gas mark 3. Line a 23cm square cake tin with baking parchment (or use a 900g loaf tin).

Put the flour, sugar, baking powder, cinnamon, bananas, figs and half the walnuts into a large bowl. Add the oil and eggs and mix well to combine. Tip the mix into the lined tin. Scatter over the remaining walnuts and seeds. Bake for 40 minutes.

Cool on a wire rack and cut into squares. Pack up for snacking on the go. Serve with peanut butter and banana or cherries and yogurt.

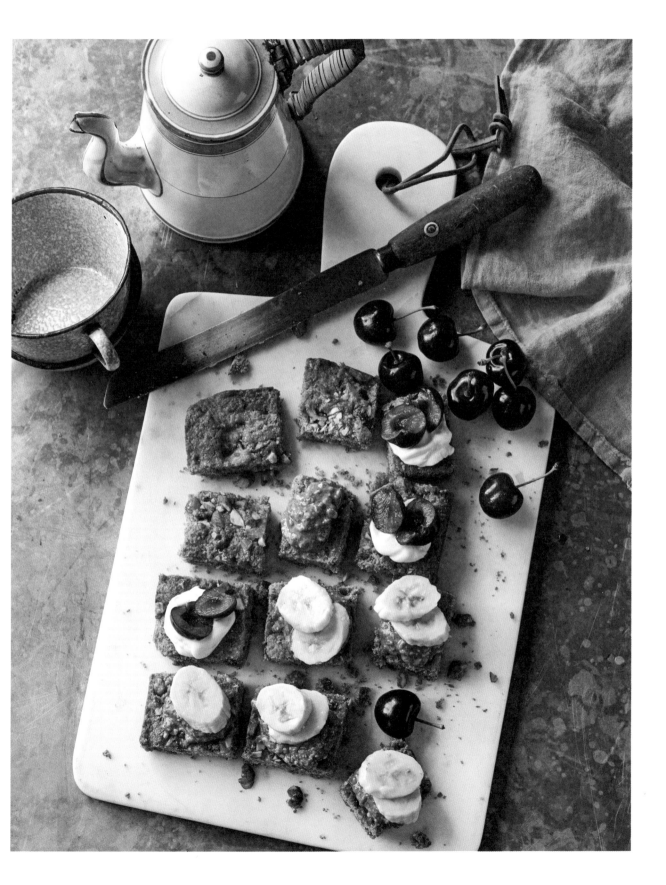

Blueberry, cashew & cacoa powerballs

serves 6

150g cashew nuts, roughly
chopped, plus
2 tablespoons finely
chopped for coating
150g blueberries
1cm piece of fresh ginger,
peeled and grated
1 tablespoon cacao
powder
1 tablespoon cacao butter
1 teaspoon coconut sugar
50g dark chocolate
(approx. 80% cocoa
solids)
1 tablespoon coconut oil

Sweet and savoury, these are the perfect snack to enjoy
with a cup of tea for an energy boost.

Blitz together the blueberries and cashew nuts in a food
processor or high-speed blender. Add the cacao powder,
coconut butter and the coconut sugar and mix together
well. Put in fridge to firm up

When firm roll into approx. 10 balls.

Melt the chocolate in a heatproof bowl set over a
saucepan of barely simmering water. Leave to cool slightly
then mix in the coconut oil.

Dip the balls into the melted chocolate, then sprinkle over
the cashews. Refrigerate or freeze. They will keep for up to
4 days in the fridge and 2 weeks in the freezer.

Nutty, seedy snack bars

makes 16

3 tablespoons raw honey
3 tablespoons coconut oil
100g rolled oats
100g mixed seeds, such as
pumpkin, sunflower and
sesame, soaked
1½ tablespoons cacao powder
50g raisins or other dried
fruit, chopped

Energy dense with good fats and glucose, these bars
make a great pre-workout snack.

Preheat the oven to 180°C/gas mark 4. Heat the honey and
coconut oil gently just to melt, then leave to cool slightly.

Tip into a bowl and mix in the oats, seeds, cocoa and
chopped fruit. Press into a small 20cm square tin. Bake for
20 minutes until firm on the top. Cool then cut into squares.

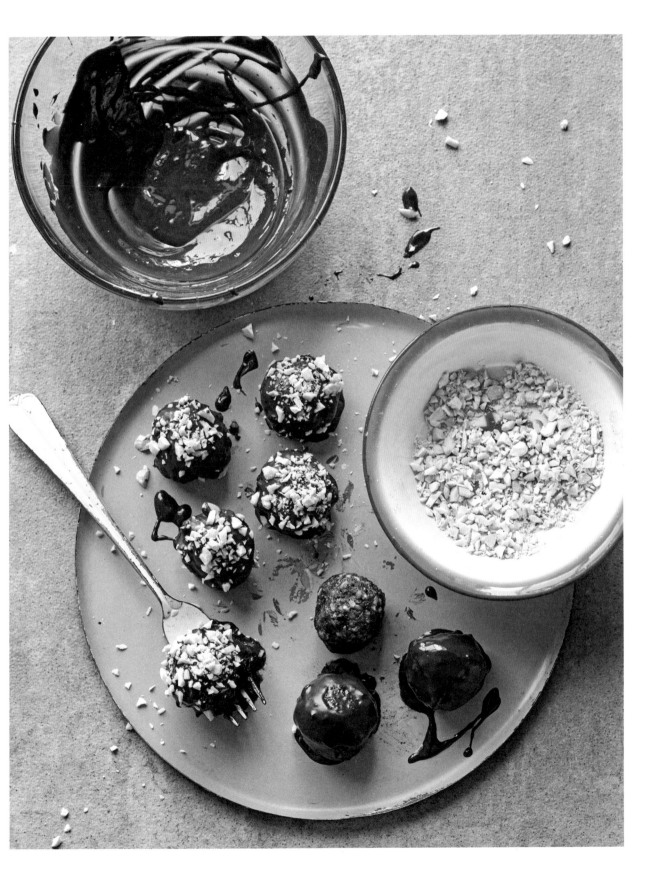

Walnut, cranberry & orange protein balls

makes 16

50g desiccated coconut,
    plus 60g toasted
2 tablespoons chia seeds
zest and juice of 1 orange
200g walnuts
175g dried cranberries
35g brown rice protein
    powder
2 tablespoons maple syrup
runny honey

Sweet and zesty, these protein balls are delicious and filling, making them a great snack to enjoy on the go.

Put the desiccated coconut and chia seeds in a bowl with the orange zest and juice. Leave for 2–3 hours for the coconut and seeds to absorb the juice.

Blitz the walnuts, cranberries, coconut and chia mix and protein powder together in a food processor.

Transfer the mixture into a bowl, add the maple syrup and knead until it is all combined and starts to stick together.

Roll level tablespoons of the mixture into 16 balls. Put a little honey onto your clean hands and roll each ball to coat in honey, then roll in the toasted desiccated coconut.

Chill for 1 hour to firm. They will keep for a couple of days in the fridge.

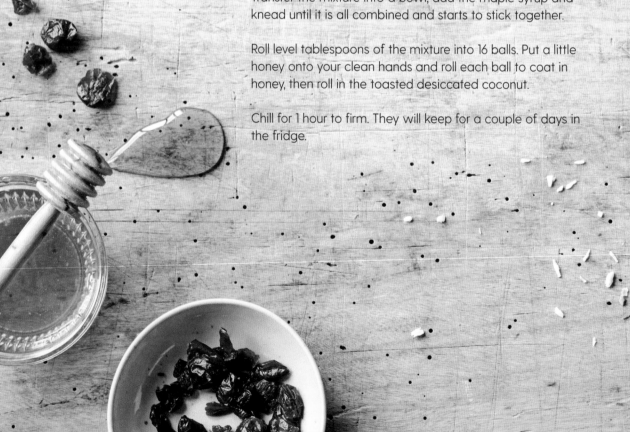

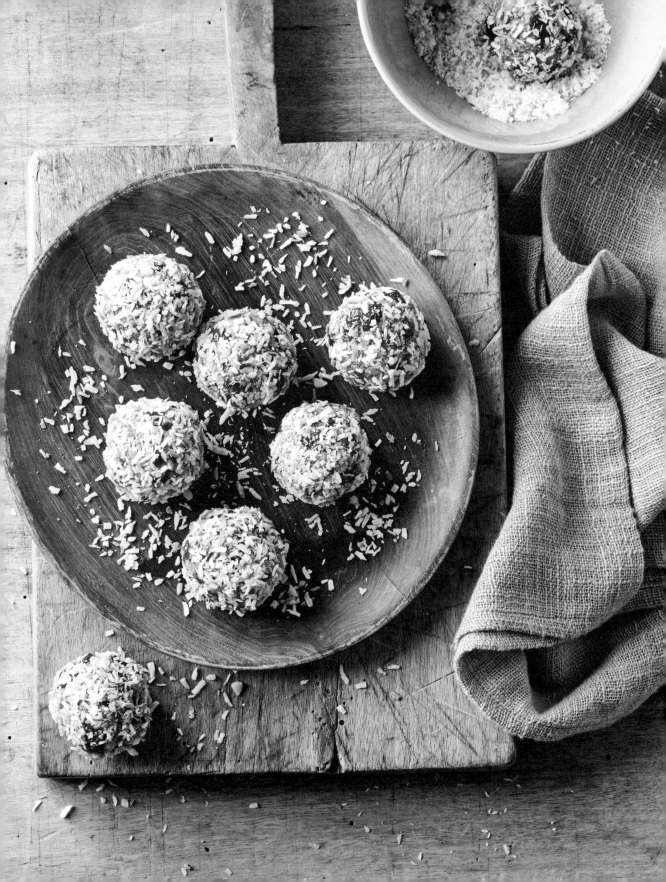

Delicious dips

CANNELLINI BEAN DIP
Serves 2–4

1 x 400g can cannellini beans, drained and rinsed

3 roasted red peppers, (from a jar in oil), drained

3 tablespoons tahini

1 garlic clove, crushed

1 teaspoon sweet smoked paprika

a handful of flat-leaf parsley, roughly chopped

50g toasted almonds

10 cherry tomatoes

sea salt and freshly ground black pepper

flatbreads or crudités, to serve

Whizz together the beans, peppers, tahini, garlic, paprika, parsley, almonds and tomatoes in a food processor or blender.

Season to taste and serve with flatbread or crudités.

AUBERGINE, MINT & LEMON DIP
Serves 2

2 large aubergines

100g cherry tomatoes, diced

2 garlic cloves, peeled

1 tablespoon Greek yogurt

a handful of mint, finely chopped

juice of 1 lemon

3 tablespoons olive oil

sea salt and freshly ground black pepper

flatbreads or crudités, to serve

Preheat the oven to 220°C/ gas mark 7:

Put the aubergines onto a roasting tray and cook until softened and the skin is lightly charred. Transfer to a colander over a bowl to drain any juices.

When cool enough to handle, peel the aubergines, then chop the flesh into a bowl. Mix in the tomatoes, garlic, yogurt, mint, lemon juice and olive oil. Season to taste and serve with flatbread or crudités.

SPICED HUMMUS
Serves 2–4

2 tablespoons olive oil

2 shallots, finely sliced into rings

1 x 400g can chickpeas, drained and rinsed

6 tablespoons tahini

2 garlic cloves, peeled

1 teaspoon ground turmeric

½ teaspoon cumin seeds, toasted and ground

juice of 1–2 lemons (to taste)

60ml cold water

2 tablespoons chopped fresh coriander

sea salt and freshly ground black pepper

flatbreads or crudités, to serve

Heat 1 tablespoon of the oil in a frying pan and sauté the shallots over a very low heat until soft and golden.

In a food processor or blender, whizz together the chickpeas, tahini, garlic, spices, lemon juice, water, half the shallots and coriander. Season to taste.

Serve the hummus topped with the remaining fried shallots and a drizzle of oil.

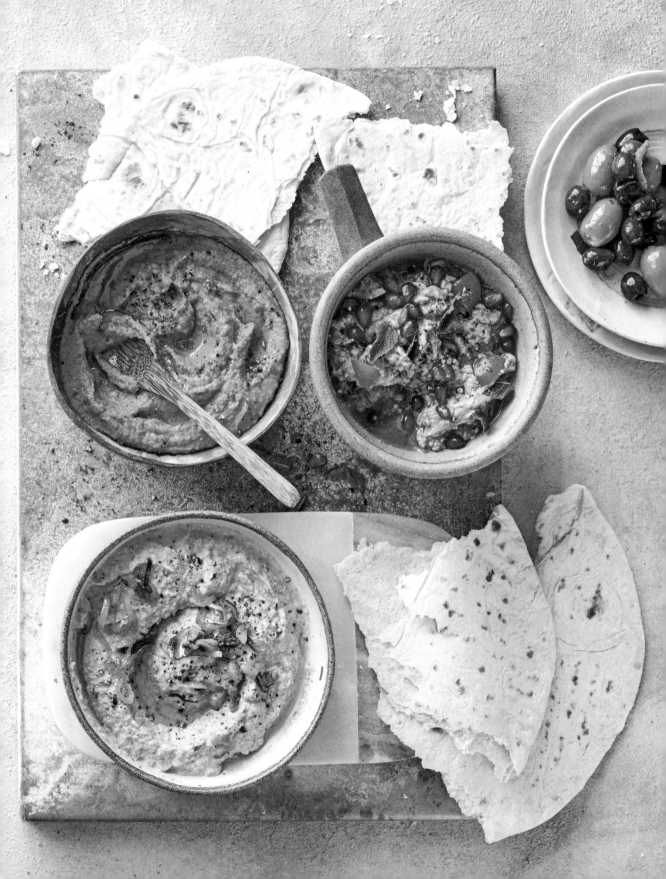

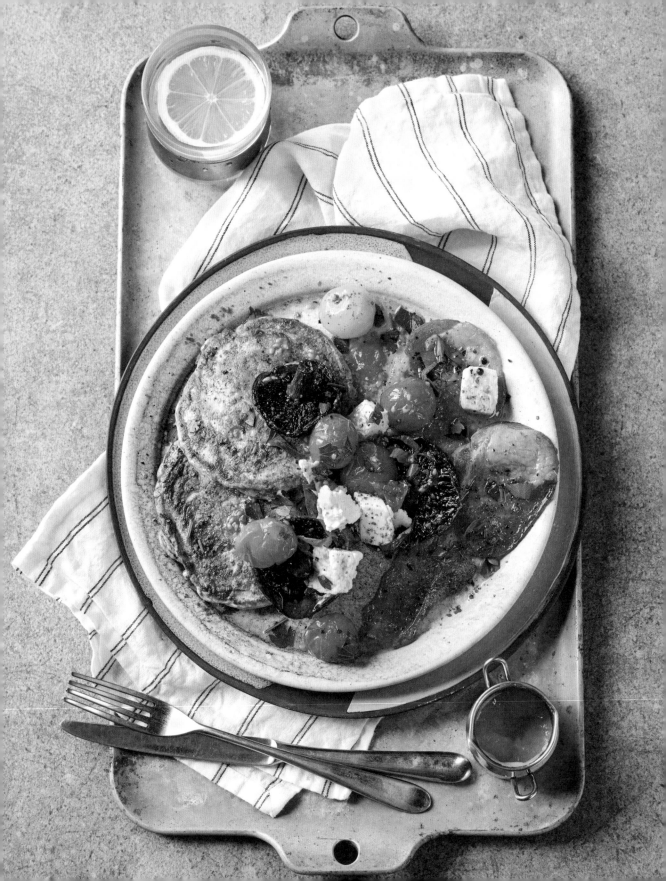

Spinach & herb pancakes with bacon, roast mushrooms & cherry tomatoes

makes 10-12 pancakes

150g cherry tomatoes

8 slices unsmoked back bacon

12 portobellini mushrooms

150g white spelt or plain flour

2 teaspoons baking powder

2 eggs, lightly whisked

200ml buttermilk or milk

50g baby leaf spinach, finely chopped

5 tablespoons chopped flat-leaf parsley, plus extra to serve

olive oil or butter, for frying

sea salt and freshly ground pepper

TO SERVE

100g cheese, such as feta or grated mature Cheddar (*optional*)

English mustard

The addition of greens to these pancakes gives them a nutritional burst of vitamins, antioxidants and minerals. Spelt flour has a lovely nutty flavour and a higher protein content than regular plain flour. Use half wholegrain spelt if you'd like the added fibre and just leave out the bacon for a veggie brunch.

Place the tomatoes, bacon and mushrooms on a lined grill pan and grill until the tomatoes and mushrooms are cooked through and the bacon is golden. Cover and keep warm while you make the pancakes.

Mix together the flour, baking powder and some seasoning. Make a well in the centre of the mixture and pour in the beaten eggs and buttermilk. Whisk well to combine. Fold through the chopped spinach and parsley. (The mix should hold in the pan so should not be too runny.)

Melt a little butter in or add a drizzle of olive oil to a large pan. For each pancake, add 2 tablespoons of mixture, making 4–6 pancakes at a time, depending on the size of your pan. Flip over when golden and little bubbles appear on the surface. Cook until golden on the other side.

Serve 2–3 pancakes with the grilled goodies and the cheese, if you wish. Finish with some chopped parsley and serve with mustard.

RUNNING LIFE

Lentils, quinoa & spinach bowl

serves 4

---

2 tablespoons olive oil
1 large shallot, chopped
2 large carrots, peeled and
    cut into large dice
250g mushrooms, roughly
    chopped
3 garlic cloves, crushed
1 teaspoon chilli flakes
1 teaspoon dried oregano
1 sprig fresh of rosemary,
    chopped
2 sprigs of thyme, leaves
    picked
1 bay leaf
1 teaspoon cumin seeds,
    toasted and ground
200g red lentils
250ml vegetable stock
360ml water
125g red quinoa or variety of
    your choice
150g spinach
sea salt and freshly ground
    black pepper

TO SERVE
olive oil
fresh herbs (*optional*)
chopped cashew nuts

A delicious vegan bowl to enjoy for a plant-based lunch or light dinner. Spinach is an excellent source of vitamins K, A, B, B6, E and C as well as choline, an important antioxidant. The quinoa and lentils provide the protein.

Heat the oil over a medium heat in a large saucepan or pot. Add the shallot and carrots and cook for 3–4 minutes until the carrots have started to soften. Add the mushrooms and continue to cook for a further 5 minutes until they are juicy and tender.

Add the garlic, chilli flakes, dried and fresh herbs and ground cumin. Stir for about a minute until the whole mixture becomes fragrant.

Pour in the lentils, stock and 225ml water. Bring to the boil, cover and simmer for 15 minutes.

Remove the lid and add the quinoa and remaining water. Stir to combine. Return to the boil, re-cover and reduce to a simmer. Cook for about 15 minutes until the lentils and quinoa are tender. Add a little more water if necessary. It will thicken as it cooks and the lentils break down.

Remove the pan from the heat, uncover and add the spinach, stirring gently to combine. Season to taste with salt and pepper.

Serve with a drizzle of olive oil, fresh herbs and chopped cashew nuts.

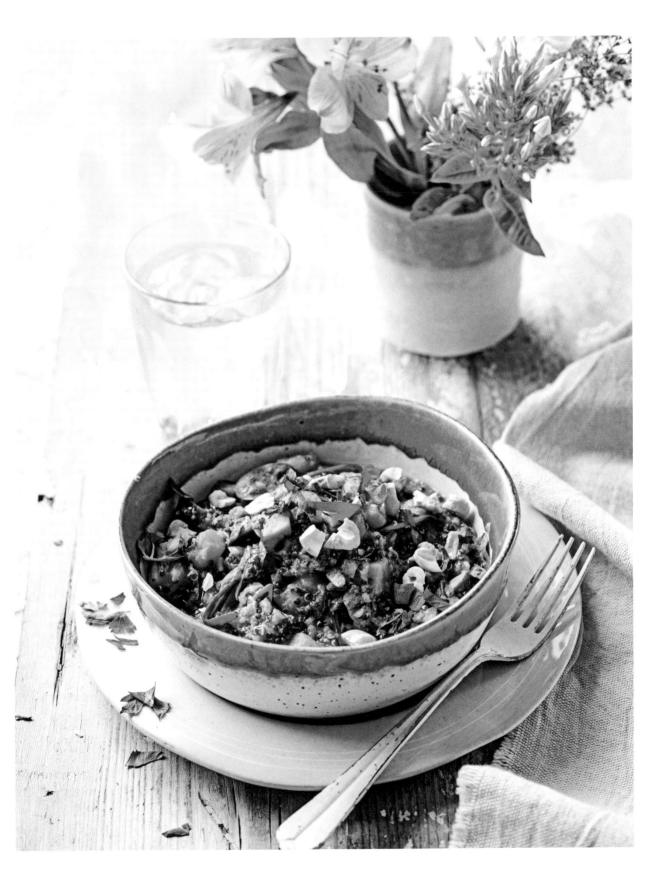

Veggie quesadillas with cheese

serves 4

1 small butternut squash, peeled and cubed (350g peeled flesh)

1 large onion, finely chopped

1 red pepper, deseeded, sliced

2 tablespoons olive oil or coconut oil, melted

2 garlic cloves, finely chopped

1 teaspoon cumin seeds, toasted and ground

1 teaspoon coriander seeds, toasted and ground

½ teaspoon smoked paprika

400g tomato rustica

1–2 teaspoons chipotle chilli paste (to taste)

2 x 400g cans black beans, drained and rinsed

sea salt and freshly ground black pepper

4 tortilla wraps or flatbreads

100g cheese of your choice, such as feta, mature Cheddar or grilled halloumi

4 tablespoons thick Greek or natural yogurt

FOR THE SALSA

1 large, ripe avocado, cubed

a handful of fresh coriander, chopped

2 chillies, deseeded and chopped

zest and juice of 1–2 limes

A lovely substantial mix of sweet vegetables, spicy beans, creamy avocado and melting cheese. Protein, carbs, fibre and healthy fats all in one. Add grilled chicken or steak if you need some extra protein. For variety, you could serve with wholegrain rice instead of the wraps or swap Skyr for the natural yogurt for a higher protein option. A great meal to enjoy after training.

Preheat the oven to 200°C/gas mark 6. Spread the squash, onion and pepper onto a roasting tray. Drizzle over half the oil, season well and roast for about 15 minutes until softened and beginning to caramelise around the edges.

Sprinkle over the garlic and spices and spoon over the tomatoes and chipotle paste. Return to the oven for a further 15 minutes. The mix should be quite thick and the vegetables cooked but not mushy. Stir through the beans and season to taste. Return to the oven for 5 minutes just to heat through.

Prepare the salsa by mixing all the ingredients together in a small bowl. Season to taste.

To serve, lay a tortilla out and spoon the bean mixture along the centre. Top with the cheese and a dollop of yogurt and salsa and roll up like a cigar or a burrito, however you find it easiest to eat! Alternatively put the bean mixture, salsa and yogurt into little piles and scoop up with flatbread.

Quinoa with harissa-spiced chickpeas

serves 2

100g mixed quinoa
1 teaspoon cumin seeds
1 tablespoon olive oil
2 shallots, finely chopped
1 fat garlic clove, finely
   chopped
2.5cm piece of fresh ginger,
   peeled and finely chopped
1 x 400g can chickpeas,
   drained and rinsed
1 tablespoon rose harissa
zest and juice of 1 lime, plus
   extra wedges to serve
a handful of fresh coriander,
   chopped
100g rocket or baby spinach
sea salt and freshly ground
   black pepper

A satisfying and balanced meal with warming, spicy flavours. Quinoa is such an adaptable grain and a great staple for many dishes. It's also easy to pre-prepare, adding last-minute ingredients and dressings depending on your mood. It's high in carbs, a good source of complete protein and contains more beneficial amounts of vitamins and minerals than most grains – namely B1, phosphorous and iron. The white variety contains slightly higher amounts than red, however red has a wonderful nutty flavour so it's good to mix it up for some variety. Toasting the grain for a couple of minutes before cooking enhances the flavour. Add grilled chicken or salmon to this dish for extra protein. A good meal to load up on macros the day before any intensive training.

Put the quinoa and cumin seeds into a pan and toast for 2–3 minutes. Add 300ml water, cover and simmer gently for 10 minutes or until the water is absorbed and the grains tender. Tip into a bowl and set aside.

Meanwhile, in another pan heat the oil and gently sauté the shallots, garlic and ginger for a few minutes to soften. Add the chickpeas, harissa, lime zest and juice and cook for a couple of minutes to infuse all the flavours.

Add the chickpeas to the quinoa along with the coriander and rocket or spinach. Season, mix well and serve with lime wedges for squeezing over the top.

Final kick wrap with spicy chilli sauce

serves 4

2 chicken breasts, cooked
1 avocado, stoned, peeled and diced
1 mango, stoned, peeled and diced
1 red chilli, finely chopped
½ teaspoon cumin seeds, toasted and ground
a handful of fresh coriander, roughly chopped
juice and zest of 1–2 limes
4 wholemeal tortilla wraps
8 crispy dolce verde leaves
4 spring onions, sliced
sea salt and freshly ground black pepper
sweet chilli sauce with a squeeze of lime juice, to serve

The red chilli and sweet chilli sauce give a tasty kick to this chicken wrap. Chicken is a great source of lean protein and contains all the essential amino acids as well as being relatively low in saturated fat compared to other animal proteins. It also provides the antioxidant selenium and vitamin B3 (niacin) responsible for converting carbohydrates to energy.

Shred the cooked chicken and set aside.

Mix together the avocado, mango, chilli, cumin, coriander and lime zest and juice.

Lay out the tortillas on a board and top with lettuce, chicken, avocado and mango salsa and spring onions. Season and drizzle with sweet chilli sauce.

Roll up like a cigar, cut in half and enjoy.

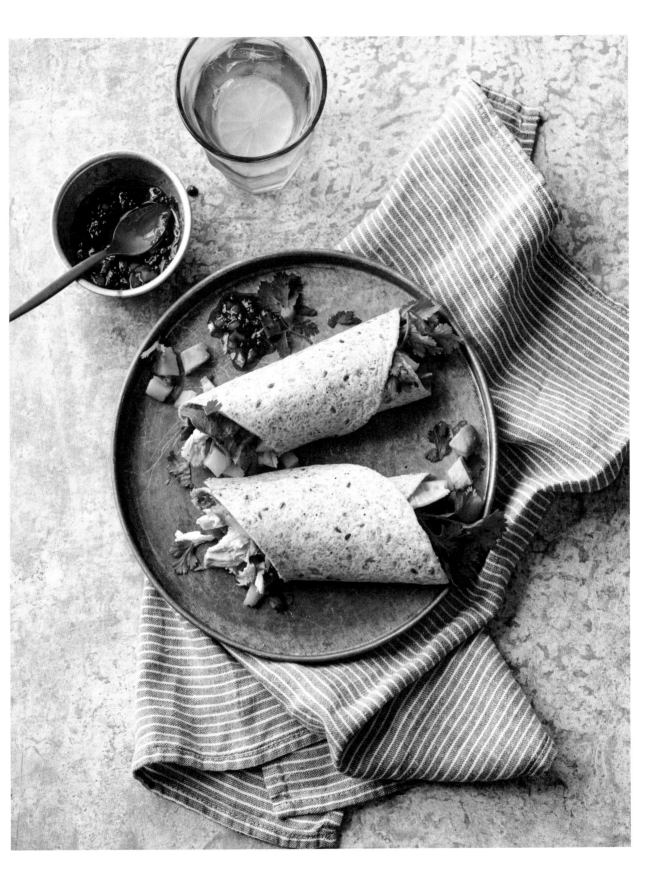

Starter's orders wrap

serves 4

---

2 sweet potatoes

1 tablespoon olive oil

2 teaspoons cumin seeds

250g pouch ready-cooked lentils of your choice, such as Puy or beluga

200g cherry tomatoes, halved

1 red pepper, deseeded and sliced

2 handfuls of spinach or mixed baby leaves

4 raw spinach tortilla wraps

sea salt and freshly ground black pepper

FOR THE PESTO

1 garlic clove

75g basil leaves

50g pine nuts

50g Parmesan, grated

150ml extra virgin olive oil

A tasty vegetarian wrap – just leave out the pesto for a vegan option. Sweet potatoes are a rich source of fibre as well as containing lots of vitamins and minerals including iron, calcium, selenium, vitamin C and most B vitamins. They're also high in the antioxidant beta-carotene which the body converts to vitamin A when eaten.

Preheat the oven to 180°C/gas mark 4.

Chop the sweet potatoes into chip shapes and spread out onto a roasting tray. Drizzle over the olive oil and scatter over the cumin seeds. Season and roast for 25 minutes until beginning to caramelise around the edges.

Put the ingredients for the pesto into a small food processor (or chop by hand). Pulse to chop, leaving some texture.

Lay out the roast sweet potatoes, lentils, tomatoes, red pepper, leaves and pesto alongside the wraps and make up the wraps as you wish.

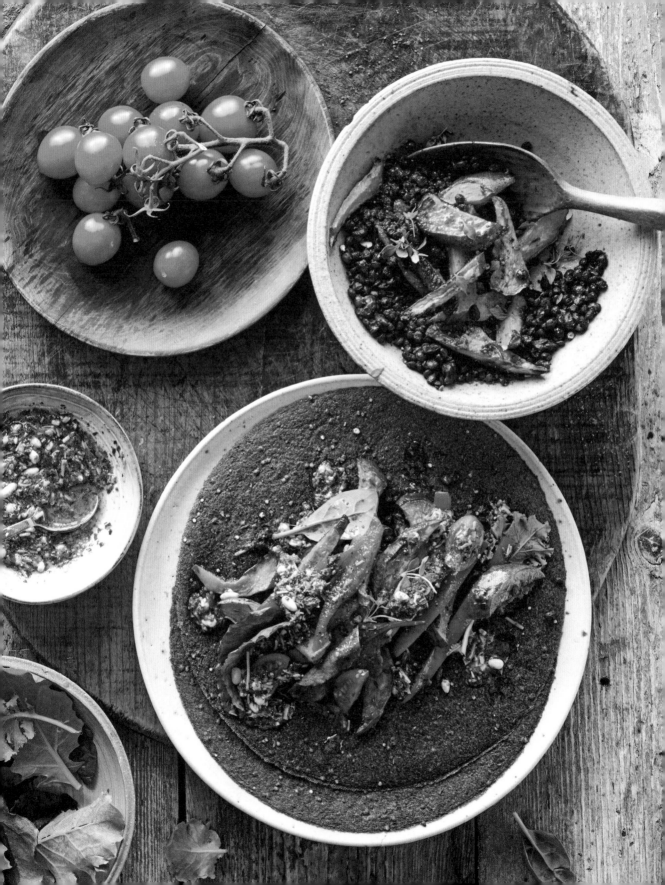

Pomegranate, kale & butter bean salad

serves 2-3

150g brown rice
1 tablespoon olive oil
200g kale, roughly chopped
1 tablespoon ground cumin
1 x 400g can butter beans, drained and rinsed
100g pomegranate seeds
2 teaspoons ground coriander
sea salt and freshly ground black pepper

FOR THE DRESSING
zest and juice of ½ orange
zest and juice 1 lemon
1 fat garlic clove, crushed
1cm piece of fresh ginger, peeled and grated
5 tablespoons extra virgin olive oil

This salad makes a great portable lunch to take to work. The kale and pomegranate are both rich in vitamins A and C as well as calcium and potassium. The pomegranate is also a good source of iron while the kale provides extra vitamins B6, B1, B2 and E as well as niacin.

Cook the brown rice in boiling water for 20–25 minutes. Drain and leave to cool.

Meanwhile, heat the olive oil in a saucepan over a medium heat and stir-fry the kale to wilt.

Sprinkle the cumin over the kale, season and leave to cool.

Mix with the butter beans, rice, pomegranate seeds and ground coriander.

Mix together all the ingredients for the dressing in a small bowl. Pour over the salad, toss well and season to taste.

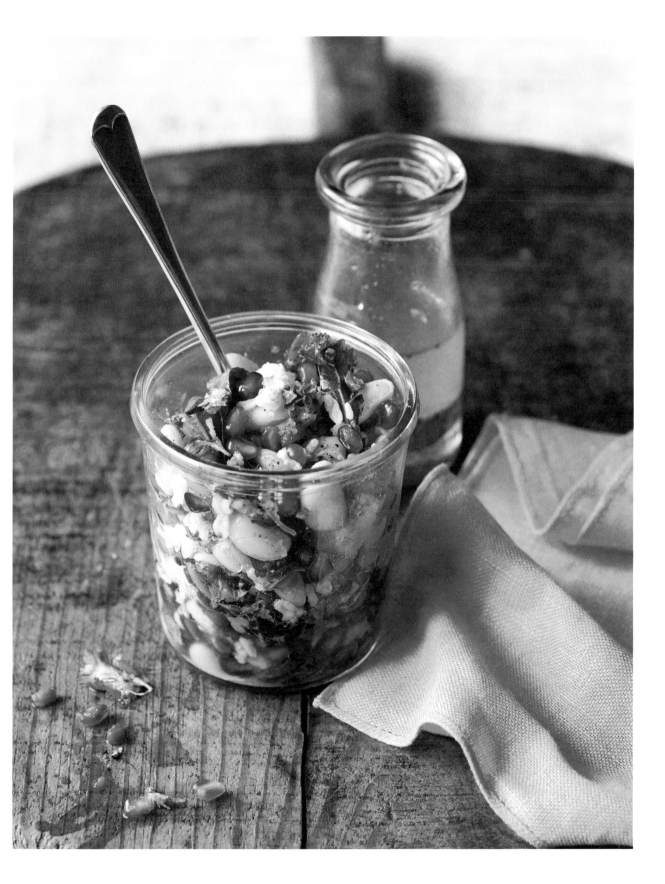

Thai chicken salad with mango & chilli dressing

serves 2

2 teaspoons coconut oil

2 organic chicken breasts
(skin off or on as you
prefer)

dash of soy sauce or tamari

3 tablespoons roasted
cashews or peanuts,
roughly chopped and extra
sliced chilli (*optional*)

FOR THE DRESSING

30ml lemon juice

1 tablespoon Thai fish sauce

finely grated zest and
juice of 3 limes

1 ripe mango, stoned, peeled
and roughly chopped

5cm piece of fresh ginger,
peeled and grated

2 chillies, deseeded and
chopped

2 tablespoons chopped fresh
coriander

sea salt and freshly ground
black pepper

FOR THE SALAD

1 dolce verde or romaine
lettuce, leaves torn

4 spring onions, finely sliced

1 carrot, peeled and shredded

1 sweet pepper, deseeded
and very thinly sliced

a handful of both fresh
coriander and mint leaves

A fresh-tasting, power-packed, protein-rich salad that is full of fibre to aid blood sugar control. Add wholegrain rice on the side for some slow energy-releasing carbs. Mangoes are a powerhouse of nutrients; they're packed with vitamins (C and B). All good brain foods here! This dish also provides calcium and vitamin K2 for bone health, and antioxidants, such as quercetin, zeaxanthin, astragalin and beta-carotene, which are all essential for cellular repair. A great meal to include in your run up to training.

Put the ingredients for the dressing into high-speed blender or food processor and blend until smooth. Season and set aside.

Heat the oil in a pan and sear the chicken on both sides until golden, seasoning as you go. Cover and cook for 5 minutes. Add a dash of soy sauce, re-cover and remove from the heat. Set aside for 5 minutes – the residual heat will cook the chicken perfectly. Cool slightly, then slice thinly on the diagonal.

Put all the salad ingredients apart from the herbs into a bowl, add half the dressing, mix well, then divide between two bowls. Top with the chicken and herbs and the roasted nuts and chilli, if using. Serve with the dressing drizzled over the top.

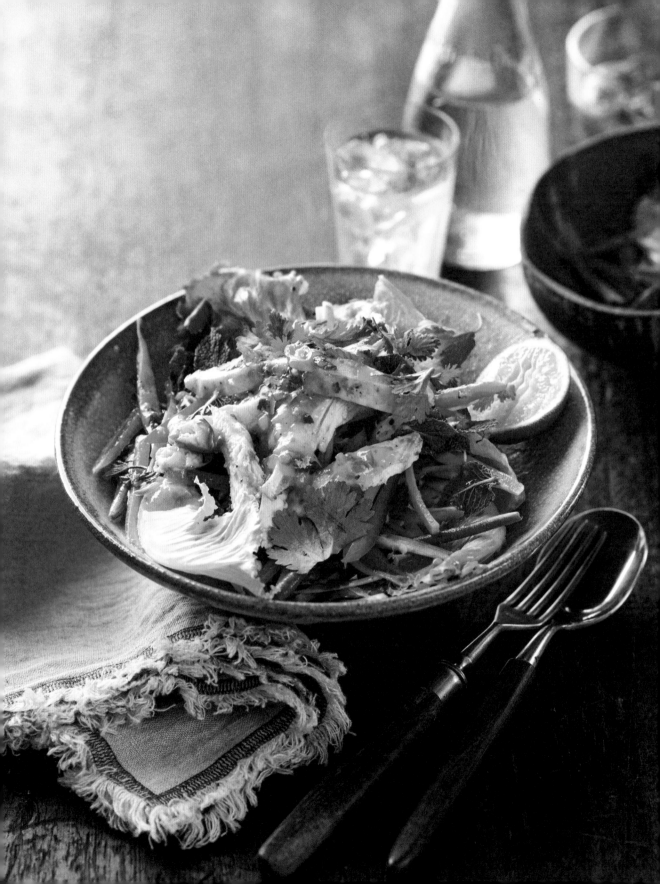

Soy, star anise & ginger baked mackerel

serves 2

5cm piece of fresh ginger, peeled and julienned

1 garlic clove, crushed

3 star anise

50ml light soy sauce

½ teaspoon light muscovado sugar

2 tablespoons sesame oil

2 mackerel fillets

2 sweet potatoes, cut into chunky chips

1 teaspoon dulse seaweed flakes (*optional*)

100g fine green beans, broccoli or kale

sea salt and freshly ground black pepper

Mackerel is an omega-3-rich fish and is also cheap, quick and easy to prepare. Make sure you get the freshest fish from your fishmonger who can also fillet it for you. Sweet potatoes are a great source of complex carbs; loaded with beta-carotene they also have antioxidant and anti-inflammatory properties. Seaweed is a dense source of vitamins and minerals. Eat with greens of your choice for a perfectly balanced pre- or post-workout meal.

Preheat the oven to 200°C/gas mark 6. Mix together the ginger, garlic, star anise, soy sauce, sugar and 1 tablespoon of the sesame oil. Pour the mixture over the mackerel in a dish and leave to marinate for 30 minutes.

Put the sweet potatoes onto a roasting tray and drizzle with the remaining sesame oil. Season with pepper. Cook for 30 minutes or until beginning to caramelise around the edges. Remove from the oven. Sprinkle over the seaweed flakes, if using, and keep warm.

Turn the oven onto grill. (Or Increase the oven to 220°C/gas mark 7 if you don't have an oven/grill combo.) Remove the fish from the marinade and place skin-side up in a snug roasting tray lined with foil; you don't want all the juices to run away and dry up. Season and cook for 6–8 minutes until the skin is beginning to crisp and the fish is just cooked through. Cover with foil and leave to sit for 5 minutes while you steam the beans.

Steam the beans for 3 minutes or just long enough to retain some crunch. Serve together with the mackerel and roast sweet potatoes and any pan juices poured over the top.

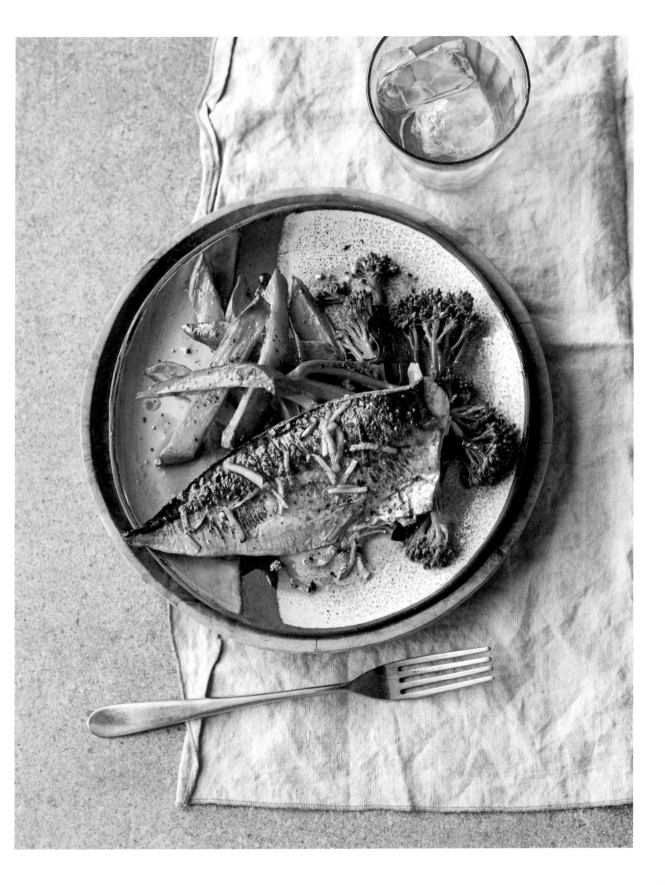

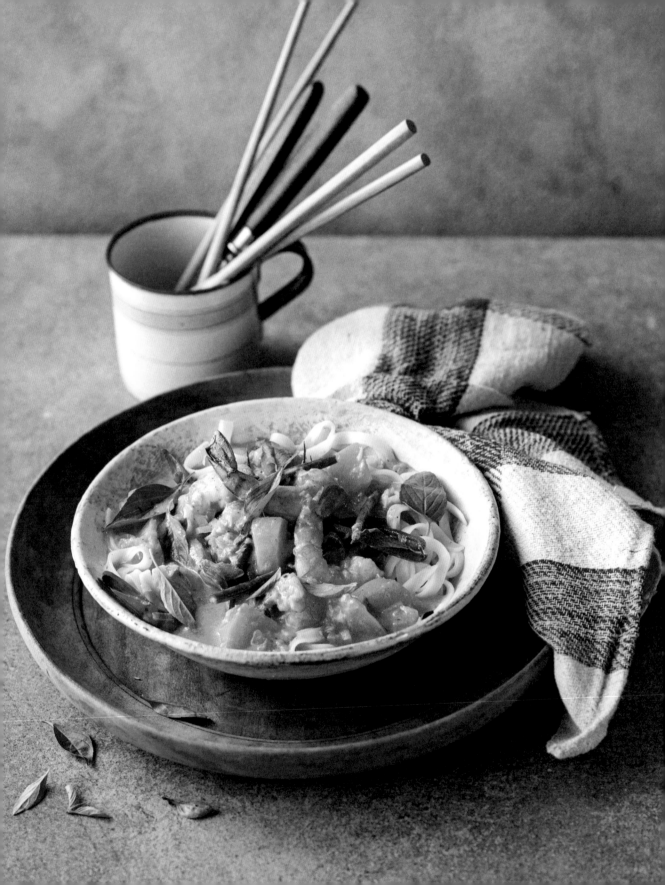

Prawn, squash & spinach Thai curry

serves 4

2 teaspoons sesame oil

4 banana shallots, sliced

3cm piece of fresh ginger, peeled and grated

2 fat garlic cloves, crushed

3 chillies, deseeded and finely chopped

4 lime leaves

2 sticks of lemongrass, bashed

5 juicy tomatoes, chopped

1 x 400ml can coconut milk

1 tablespoon crunchy peanut butter

350g butternut squash, peeled and cut into chunks

20 large prawns, peeled and deveined

100g baby spinach

100g fine green beans

zest and juice of 1 lime

sea salt and freshly ground black pepper.

rice noodles or rice, to serve

a handful of Thai basil (*optional*)

A warming, nourishing curry to be enjoyed post-workout, when relaxing or the evening before a training session to stock up on your macronutrients. Handfuls of spinach, barely cooked, are a great source of iron and antioxidants. Always have some citrus with iron-rich foods, either lemon juice squeezed over the top, as in this dish, or squeezed into water to drink alongside. It renders the iron far more bioavailable. The prawns can be substituted for salmon, chicken or tofu.

Heat the oil in a saucepan and sauté the shallots until translucent. Add the ginger, garlic and chillies and cook for a few minutes until fragrant. Add the lime leaves, lemongrass, tomatoes, coconut milk, 400ml water and the peanut butter. Simmer for 5 minutes. Add the butternut squash and cook until just tender, but still has a little bite.

Add the prawns and simmer very gently for 5 minutes until pink and just cooked through. Add the spinach, green beans, lime zest and juice, then stir well and leave for 5 minutes for all the flavours to infuse. Season to taste.

Serve with rice noodles or rice, a scattering of Thai basil and chilli, if you like.

Chicken wrapped in bacon with lemon & mustard broccoli

serves 2

100g tenderstem broccoli
2 teaspoons olive oil
2 skinless chicken breasts
4 slices of streaky bacon or
   pancetta
75g cracked freekeh, soaked
   in water for 5 minutes
   then drained or 250g pack
   ready-prepared freekeh or
   other grain of your choice,
   such as Puy lentils or
   quinoa
150ml light chicken stock
a large handful of kale,
   shredded
2 tablespoons capers,
   drained
a large handful of flat-leaf
   parsley, roughly chopped
25g pumpkin seeds, toasted
sea salt and freshly ground
   black pepper

FOR THE DRESSING
1 fat garlic clove, crushed
zest and juice of 1 lemon
1 heaped teaspoon English
   mustard
4 tablespoons extra virgin
   olive oil

Freekeh is a deliciously earthy, nutty grain. It has a good nutritional profile being low fat, higher in protein than other grains and very high in fibre, vitamins and iron. It also has prebiotic benefits which help maintain a healthy digestive system.

Preheat the oven to 220°C/gas mark 7. Mix together the ingredients for the dressing and set aside.

Put the broccoli onto a roasting tray, season and drizzle with 1 teaspoon of oil. Wrap two slices of bacon around each chicken breast.

Heat 1 teaspoon of oil in a pan and brown the chicken on all sides. Season. place on top of the broccoli then transfer to the oven for 10 minutes. The chicken should be just cooked through and the broccoli softened and lightly charred around the edges. Remove the chicken and broccoli from the oven and pour over the dressing.

Tip the freekeh into a saucepan and add the stock. Cover and simmer gently for 15 minutes until the stock has almost been absorbed. (If using ready-cooked grains, add to a saucepan with 100ml boiling water and cook for 3–4 minutes.) Add the kale, cover and cook for a further 5 minutes until the kale wilts. Add the capers and season.

Slice the chicken and serve with the broccoli, freekeh and a sprinkling of parsley and pumpkin seeds.

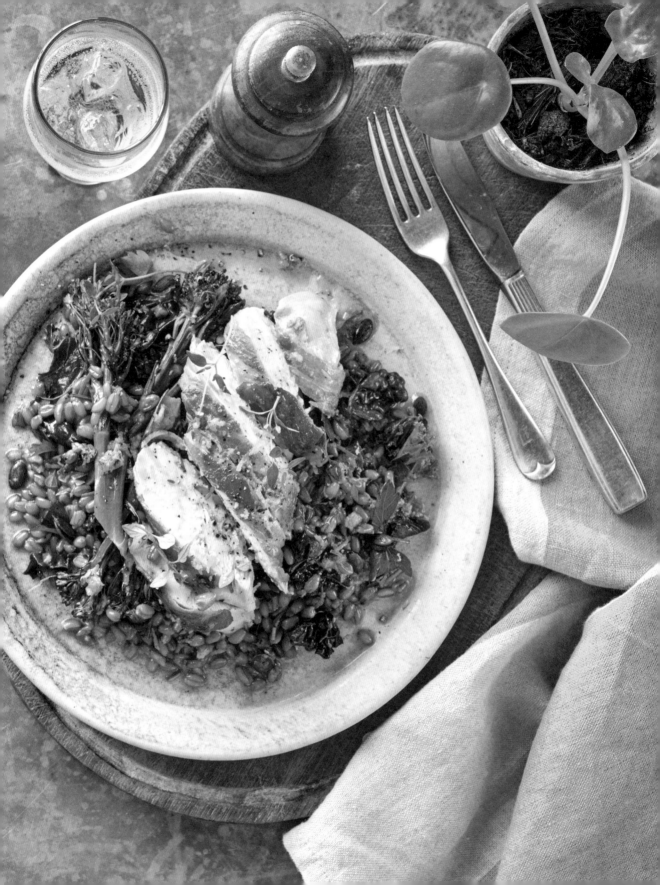

A really good dhal

serves 4

3 tablespoons coconut oil

2 large onions, finely
  chopped

1 heaped teaspoon cumin
  seeds

4 garlic cloves, finely
  chopped

5cm piece of fresh ginger,
  peeled and finely chopped

1 teaspoon coriander seeds,
  crushed

1 teaspoon Ceylon ground
  cinnamon

3 teaspoons ground turmeric

½ teaspoon asafoetida

200g chana dhal, soaked
  in 750ml water overnight,
  drained and rinsed

1.25 litres vegetable stock

200g red lentils

2 sweet potatoes, peeled and
  cut into bite-size chunks

1 x 400ml can coconut milk

10 curry leaves (*optional*)

150g spinach

sea salt and freshly ground
  black pepper

TO SERVE

a bunch of fresh coriander,
  roughly chopped

2 chillies, finely chopped
  (*optional*)

Eaten with rice this dish provides all the essential amino acids. In addition to providing nutrients, coconut milk contains a beneficial fat called lauric acid, a medium chain fatty acid which can help stimulate your metabolism. What's more it is easily absorbed and used by the body as energy rather than stored as fat (noting of course that energy intake does not exceed energy expenditure). The addition of anti-inflammatory spices and nutrient-rich vegetables make it a perfect pre- or post-training meal.

Heat the oil in a pan and add the onions and cumin. Cook for 8–10 minutes until softened and golden. Add the garlic, ginger and coriander seeds and cook for a further couple of minutes.

Add the cinnamon, turmeric, asafoetida, chana dhal and stock and bring to the boil. Reduce the heat and simmer for 30–45 minutes until the dhal is almost tender (this will differ between brands and how long the dried dhal has been on the shelf).

Add the red lentils, sweet potatoes, coconut milk and curry leaves and continue cooking for 20–25 minutes until the sauce is reduced, the dhal and potatoes are completely tender and the red lentils are beginning to break down. (Stir every so often and top up with water if the dhal is looking at all dry.)

Season to taste and stir through the spinach to wilt. Serve with coriander and the chopped chilli, if you wish.

Quinoa & lentil burgers

serves 6

100g green lentils

100g red quinoa

1 large sweet potato, peeled and cut into chunks

1 tablespoon olive oil, plus extra for frying

1 onion, finely chopped

1 large carrot, peeled and grated

2 garlic cloves, finely chopped

1 teaspoon ground cumin

½ teaspoon mild chilli powder

a small handful of fresh coriander, chopped

30g cashews, roasted and finely chopped

75–100g panko breadcrumbs

6 slices of mature Cheddar cheese

6 wholegrain buns or large lettuce leaves

sea salt and freshly ground black pepper

TO SERVE

crispy lettuce, sliced tomato, pickles, onion marmalade, sliced jalapeños, sliced sautéed field mushrooms, ketchup, mayonnaise

Together with the vegetables, nuts and lentils these quinoa burgers are a protein-packed feast. Have on half a bun with lots of salad if you'd like to reduce your refined carb load. You can also oven-bake these burgers with a drizzle of olive oil, but they taste better fried. Allowed every once in a while!

Cook the lentils in boiling water for 15–20 minutes until tender but not mushy. Drain well.

Meanwhile, put the quinoa in another pan with 300ml water, cover and cook for 15 minutes until tender. The quinoa should soak up all the water. Leave to cool slightly then tip into a bowl with the lentils. Steam the sweet potato until just tender, then crush with a fork and mix with the quinoa and lentils.

Heat the oil in a pan and cook the onion and carrot for about 10 minutes until really soft and beginning to caramelise. Add the garlic, cumin and chilli powder and cook for a further couple of minutes. Tip into the bowl with the quinoa, lentils and sweet potato, add the coriander and cashews and season really well.

Tip the panko breadcrumbs into a shallow bowl. Divide the burger mixture into 6 balls and squeeze each together really well to make patties. Dip the patties into the panko, pressing the breadcrumbs into the sides. Put them into the fridge to firm up for at least 1 hour.

When ready to cook, heat a large glug of oil in a roomy pan. Fry the patties until golden on each side and heated through. Pop a slice of cheese onto the cooked side when you flip them over; the heat will melt it. Serve inside a bun or on a large lettuce leaf, with your choice of toppings and sides.

Za'atar-spiced salmon with quinoa

serves 2

---

2 salmon fillets
3 tablespoons olive oil
2 teaspoons za'atar
zest and juice of 1 lemon
100g red quinoa
1 tablespoon mixed seeds, such as sesame, pumpkin and sunflower
a dash of soy sauce or tamari
¼ cucumber, finely diced
100g cherry tomatoes, diced
3 spring onions, finely sliced
2 tablespoons Greek olives, roughly chopped
1 tablespoon capers, drained
a handful of both fresh coriander and flat-leaf parsley, finely chopped
3cm piece of fresh ginger, peeled and finely chopped
sea salt and freshly ground black pepper

In this recipe there's lots of herbs and salad veggies added to the quinoa for an extra boost of vitamins and antioxidants, plus some ginger for its anti-inflammatory benefits. You can substitute the olives and capers for 50g pomegranate seeds if you prefer. Salmon is packed with omega-3 fatty acids, which are essential for heart and brain health as well as helping to reduce inflammation. Always opt for organic or wild salmon if you have the choice. The astaxanthin content is higher in wild salmon, which gives it its red colour, and has additional free-radical-fighting antioxidant effects, so the health benefits are huge!

Preheat the grill. Season the salmon, drizzle over 1 teaspoon of oil and scatter over the za'atar and lemon zest. Grill for 6–8 minutes or until just cooked through. Squeeze over ¼ of the lemon. Cover with foil and set aside.

Toast the quinoa in a saucepan for a couple of minutes then cover in 300ml boiling water. Cook for 15 minutes until the grains are tender and beginning to split and the water has been completely absorbed. Tip into a bowl and leave to cool.

Toast the seeds in a pan over a low heat until they begin to pop a little, then shake in a little soy sauce, stir well and remove from the heat.

Add the cucumber, tomatoes, spring onions, olives, capers and herbs to the cooled quinoa. Mix together the remaining lemon juice and oil and the ginger. Stir into the quinoa, season and serve alongside the salmon.

NUTRITION

220

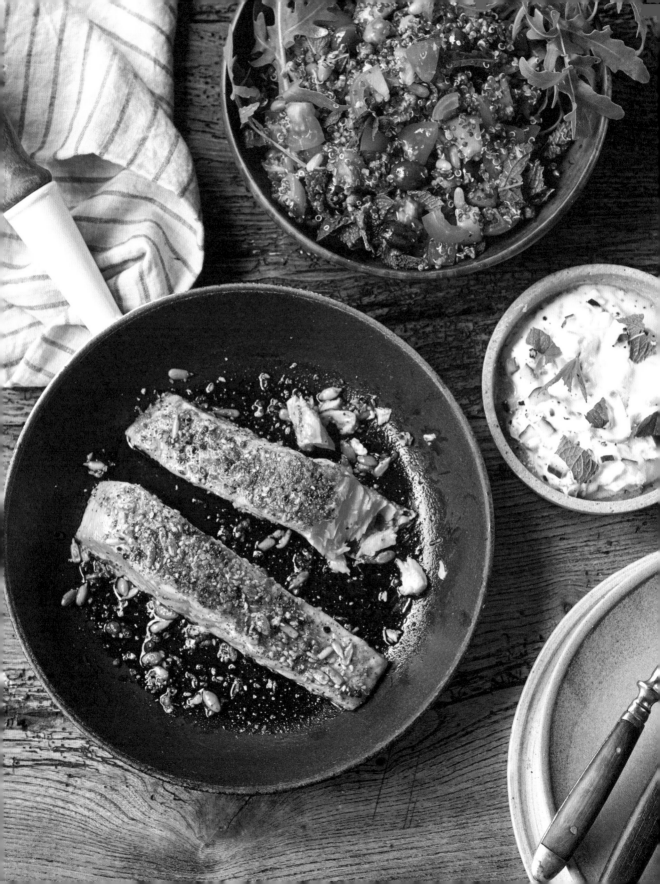

Thank you

When I started writing this book my mother was ill and because of her death I asked my publisher if they would give me time and space to get my mind straight. So my first thanks goes to Kyle Books for sticking by me, having a huge amount of patience and helping me produce a wonderful book.

The ladies and guys that have helped with the direction, your support and input has been great and our photoshoot days were a lot of fun. I want that house!

My PA Andrea, for the thousands of emails and calls with Vicky at Kyle. See you got your name in it somewhere!

I would like to thank Ali Rose who was my physio during my career and helped me to my Olympic success. Ali is a chartered physiotherapist who has been involved in sports for the last twenty years. She is also the Clinical Director for a very successful sports injury clinic in Leeds (CSPC). Since 2004, she has worked with Jessica Ennis, the 2012 Olympic heptathlon gold medallist. Ali specialises in working with sportsmen and women and has worked at the last five Olympics and numerous World and European Championships. I think she thought she had got away from me when I retired but clearly not! Our 'Flipper and Flapper' naming was a laugh.

Tanya Wright, for imparting her knowledge and helping me have a really strong Mindset section. She is a registered and accredited member of the British Association of Counselling and Psychotherapy with 10 years' experience of helping people, one-to-one and in groups. Among other things, Tanya works closely with West Kent Mind who also ran the Mental Health First Aid course that we both went on.

As I was writing this book, I had a lot of people in my mind that I have been interacting with both through social media and in person.

I want to share with you a snapshot of my life in the hope that it motivates, inspires or at least helps people to reflect. It's honest, it's real and it's me!! So here it is:
· In a children's home until I started primary school
· No privileges. Grew up in a council house and did odd jobs like cleaning cars/paper rounds/shopping for elderly to get my own money
· As a young girl I struggled with my identity because I had a white mum and grew up in a white family and didn't know my biological father (who is Jamaican)
· As a woman and a person in the public eye, I have learnt to deal with and be confident with what and who I am
· Joined the Army when I was 17 left when I was 27. Proud to have served for my country
· MBE for services to the military 1998
· Suffer from depression, self-harmed and being self-destructive
· Double Olympic champion after dreaming about it from 14 years of age
· Awarded Dame Commander of the British Empire
· Charity founder of the Dame Kelly Holmes Trust helping disadvantaged young people
· Business owner @cafe1809
· Trying to deal with bereavement because I lost my mother 2017
· Beacon award for Philanthropy 2018
· Campaigner for causes I am passionate about
· Motivational speaker
· Now honoured with the title Hon Col (Colonel)

I believe anything is possible if:

1. You are given the opportunity to achieve
2. You are given the opportunity to believe
3. You take up the opportunities that come to you
4. You never give up believing
5. You remember life is a journey. Sometimes it can be so bad that you cannot see one step in front of you and sometimes so good you can see the whole wide world available to you.

GET HELP and support if you need to
SPEAK to people because you want to
DON'T GIVE UP at the first hurdle
CRY if you have to
LOVE if you want to
DREAM because you should do

MOST OF ALL BE YOU

For all of you that buy my book, thank you. Kelly x

PICTURE CREDITS

Pages 4–5 Andy Lyons/Getty Images; page 22 (*top*) REX/Shutterstock; (*bottom right*) Kirsty Wigglesworth/ROTA/Getty Images; page 60 (*top*) Colorsport/REX/Shutterstock; page 67 (*left*) Andy Hooper/Daily Mail/REX Shutterstock; (*right*) Christopher Lee/Getty Images

Page 8 (*top and bottom right*); page 23 (*bottom left*); page 47; page 59; page 60 (*bottom left and right*); page 77 (*top left and right*); page 90 (*top left and bottom left and right*); page 122 (*top right*) courtesy of Dame Kelly Holmes @realkellyholmes1500